ONE BREATH APART
FACING DISSECTION

ONE BREATH APART
FACING DISSECTION

SANDRA L. BERTMAN
BODY DONORS AND MEDICAL STUDENTS

Foreword by **JACK COULEHAN, MD**

Designed by **DIGITALCLAY INTERACTIVE, LTD.**

Published by WARD STREET STUDIO
Newton, MA e: www.sandrabertman.com

Design: LOUISA BERTMAN.

ISBN 978-1-60461-805-1

First Edition © 2007 printed and bound by CLASSIC GRAPHX in Cambridge MA.
Second Edition © 2008 printed in China by Global PSD.

Production of this book has been made possible in part by
The ARNOLD P. GOLD FOUNDATION for HUMANISM IN MEDICINE.

SANDY C. MARKS, JR. (1937–2002)

For his mentoring, support, and friendship, this book is dedicated to the memory of Sandy C. Marks, Jr., DDS, PhD, Professor of Cell Biology, Radiology, and Surgery, and Founder of the Anatomical Gift Program at the University of Massachusetts Medical School. His vision and commitment made possible this creative collaboration, and his inspiration will continue to guide the profession not only at UMass but at medical schools throughout the world.

FOREWORD

One of the enduring images of my first year in medical school is the narrow, unshaven face of Ernest, the cadaver I shared with three classmates whose names I can't remember. We named him "Ernest," so we could impress our parents by telling them how we were working in dead earnest. In reality, like most cadavers in those days, he was an anonymous indigent man who died in the county home and whose remains were used for our education without his consent. My group was considered lucky because cancer had burned away every bit of Ernest's fat, thus making him an excellent "specimen" for dissection.

Even then I knew that Ernest was more than a specimen, but it took a long time to understand that he was actually my first mentor in the joys and sorrows and successes and failures of medicine. Surprisingly, it was Ernest rather than my basic science professors — the living ones, that is — who provoked the most important questions about what it means to be a doctor and forced me to confront them. As I recall, though, this was a solitary process because my classmates and I never discussed, or perhaps even admitted to ourselves, our feelings of ambivalence, fear, pain, gratitude, and exultation, or the changes in us as persons during the first year of medical school. We tried to hide all this because at the time that's what doctors were supposed to do.

Today things are different. Most likely if you are reading this, then you are privileged to have a module like *One Breath Apart* integrated into your anatomy experience. This module provides you the opportunity to explore and share your personal responses to dissection, and with this publication it gives you access to an additional resource: a splendid introduction to the written and visual tradition established by UMass students over the last three decades, along with evocative photographs and journal entries from the medical students at Weill Medical College of Cornell University, documented by Meryl Levin in *Anatomy of Anatomy*.

As I read through this book, I was struck by the Nancy Long's title poem. She writes, "I pretended you were here/To teach me the details." How reminiscent of my own experience those words are! "Then I saw your face/And I knew…" That's the turning point. As physicians we can either embark on the journey of learning to see others' faces and to hold their hands, or we can attempt to distance ourselves and focus only on "details." This is a decision that every medical student must make, and our cadavers present the first difficult challenge. In a 2006 class poem, UMass students wrote, "We felt the brain/And imagined its power to create. We held the heart/And imagined its ability to embrace." These words represent an affirmation of empathy and compassion over detachment.

One of the most compelling images of *One Breath Apart* shows the anatomy cadaver as a bridge spanning the chasm that lies between ignorance, darkness, and death on one side and knowledge, health, and life on the other. Dozens of tiny figures march across the span. Like me, they won't forget the backbone of that bridge. As another UMass student writes, "I know that I will be irrevocably altered."

JACK COULEHAN, MD

Dr. Jack Coulehan is a professor of medicine at Stony Brook University, where he directs the medical humanities and bioethics program. He has published four collections of poetry, most recently *Medicine Stone* (2002), and written or edited several other books, notably *The Medical Interview: Mastering Skills for Clinical Practice* (5th edition, 2006) and *Primary Care: More Poems by Physicians* (2006).

IT IS COMMONLY KNOWN THAT MEDICAL STUDENTS DISSECT THE BODIES OF THE DEAD; IT IS LESS COMMONLY REALIZED THAT THESE SAME DEAD DO A GREAT DEAL OF CUTTING, PROBING AND PULLING AT THE MINDS OF THEIR YOUTHFUL DISSECTORS.

ALAN GREGG, MD, 1957

PROLOGUE
SHARING A UMASS MEDICAL SCHOOL TRADITION

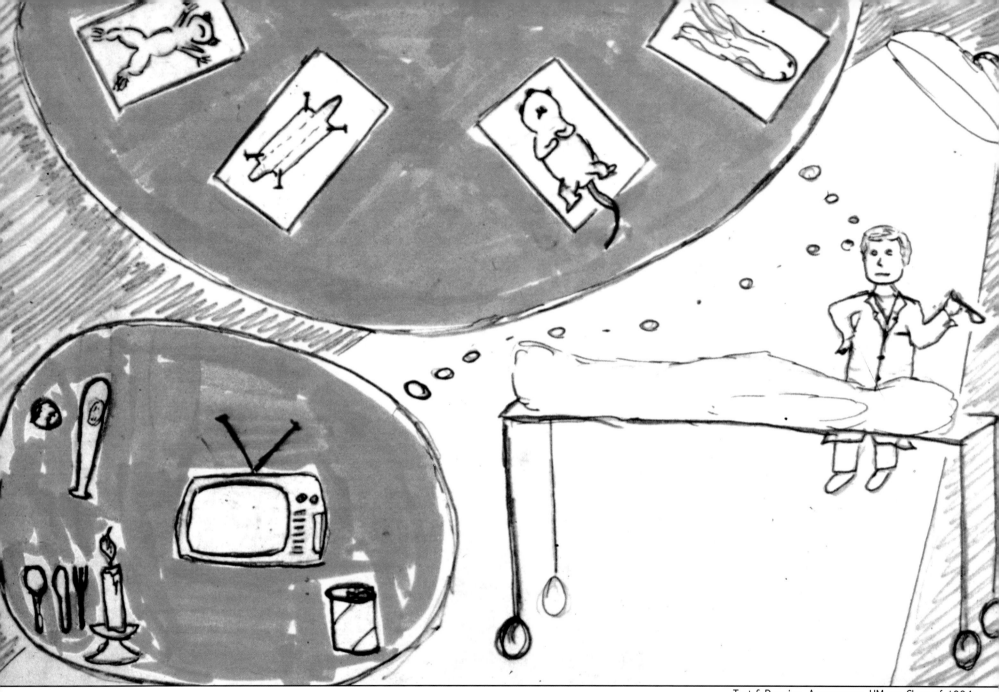

Text & Drawing, Anonymous, UMass, Class of 1994

 I've performed several dissections along the way and anticipate no problems during the human dissection. Unfortunately... I've never played baseball with a frog, eaten with an earthworm, watched a movie with a rat, nor have I gone out drinking with a squid.

First-Year Medical Student

In this book, we address you, the first-year medical student, as you face one of the most difficult hurdles in medical education — the dissection of a cadaver. A National Public Radio discussion called the anatomy course a decisive "litmus test" for how well you will fit into medicine. Occasionally this subject is explored by the mainstream media, but even then it is usually through the words of people from within the medical tradition. In the anatomy lab, author Abigail Zuger MD writes: "Every single complicated emotion anyone has ever enunciated about the practice of medicine roars into the open" (*New York Times,* July 31, 2007).

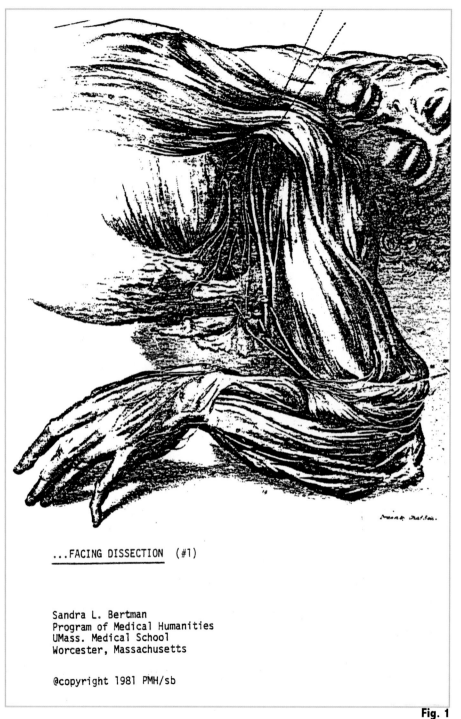

...FACING DISSECTION   (#1)

Sandra L. Bertman
Program of Medical Humanities
UMass. Medical School
Worcester, Massachusetts

@copyright 1981 PMH/sb

Fig. 1

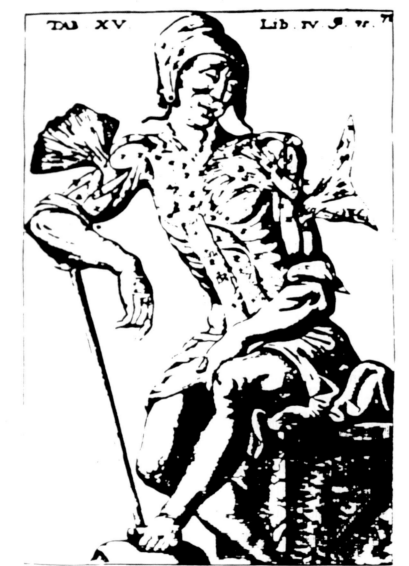

Module 1: On Death, Dying & Dissection

Sandra L. Bertman, Ph.D.
Program of Medical Humanities

Sandy C. Marks. Jr., Ph.D.
Department of Anatomy

Fall 1987

Fig. 2

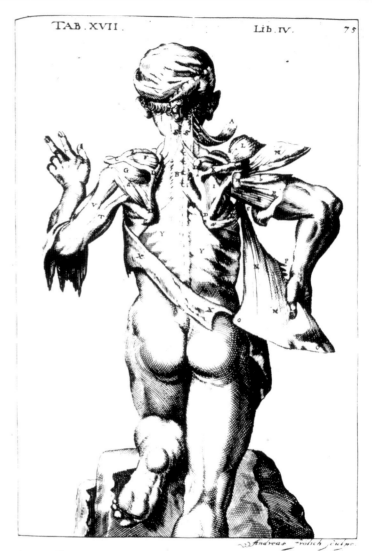

...facing dissection

On Death, Dying and Dissection

Sandra L. Bertman, Ph.D.
Program of Medical Humanities

Sandy C. Marks. Jr., Ph.D.
Department of Anatomy

Fall 1988

Fig. 3

Who lay wrapped in that sheet? What would he find when he unrolled the body and dropped the winding cloth to the floor?

Irving Stone, The Agony and the Ecstasy, 1961

DISSECTION AND REFLECTION
SIX EXPERIENCES OF THE FIRST YEAR MEDICAL STUDENTS AT UMASS

Memo: To Medical Students, Class of 2001: **Welcome!**

From: Sandra L. Bertman, Ph.D. and Sandy C. Marks, Jr., D.D.S., Ph.D.

                UMMC, Dept. of Cell Biology, Worcester, MA 01655-0802

Subject   **On Dissection, Dying and Death**

In the space below, (1) please devise an image of any sort relating to your thoughts or feelings as you anticipate the experience of dissection. (2) On the attached page, we would appreciate an explanation of your drawing or image. (3) Please mail your image and commentary to Dr. Bertman or Dr. Marks as soon as possible. We would like to incorporate these images – **anonymously**, of course,–into the presentations in August and October. See you then. Thank you.

NAME_____   Age____   Date_____

Permission granted to use my name with image in a future presentation or publication. Please circle one: (**YES**) (**NO**)

Template, Dr. Bertman   **Fig. 5**

1. Anticipating Dissection Before the Course Begins

From 1989 to 2002, students entering the University of Massachusetts Medical School were sent a blank template in the shape of a rectangular box with the invitation to reflect. The accompanying instructions read simply: "In the space provided, (1) please devise an image of any sort relating to your thoughts or feelings as you anticipate the experience of dissection. (2) On the attached page, we would appreciate an explanation of your drawing or image" (Fig. 5,6). Students were assured that their images and explanations would be used anonymously (unless permission was specifically granted to use their names).

Over the years, students responded by sketching, and cartooning, and making collages; they also commented on their drawings some seriously, others wittily, still others with dark humor, anticipating and speculating upon what dissection would be for them.

2. Inaugural Session: Facing Dissection

The three-hour Inaugural Session ("Introduction to Cell Biology") has been held on the first or second day of medical school in August of each year. The first hour is devoted to a technical description of the curriculum — what students are responsible for in their introductory course of anatomy. It is followed by an illustrated lecture: "Facing Dissection: Course Overview," conducted in partnership with the Medical Humanities faculty. The presentation delineates the history of dissection, the parallels of dissection and patient care, and the anatomical gift procedure.

Neither are graves robbed nor unclaimed bodies (criminals, paupers) pursued to provide medical students with this learning tool to master their craft. Body donors are passionate about this deliberate, altruistic act — giving their bodies for the betterment of humankind. Body donor Claire Small, at age fifty-eight, sent a personal letter to the coordinator of our Anatomical Gifts program, stating her "sense of satisfaction and fulfillment" and hoping that her message would be shared with medical, nursing, and dental students. She wrote in her letter, dated March 15, 1979: "With this modest(!) thought, I decided to send you a copy now rather than sending it only with my corpse." Accompanying her official anatomical form and letter was also a poem she had written, addressed directly to the students.

Claire Small's message has been included in the handout materials distributed to the UMass medical students at the Inaugural Session. Included in the packet have been poems such as Sylvia Plath's "Two Views of a Cadaver Room," (1960) alluding to the "panorama of smoke and slaughter" in Brueghel's painting *The Triumph of Death* (1562), as well as John Stone, MD "Cadaver"(1972), and Jack Coulehan, MD "Anatomy Lesson" (1991); the poems by these physician poets, recalling their medical school days, are particularly favored by students.

ANATOMICAL GIFT TO A MEDICAL STUDENT

THIS IS MY BODY
THE SHELL OF MY BEING
WHICH IS GIVEN TO YOU.

IN FINAL OFFERING
TO THE WORLD
I SHARE THE ELEMENTS OF LIFE.

FROM THESE OLD BONES,
THESE LIGAMENTS,
MY SINEWS AND MY NERVES
MAY THAT LIFE FORCE
THAT RAN IN ME
SHINE FORTH ONCE MORE
AND PASS TO YOU
THE KNOWLEDGE AND THE POWER
THAT HELP SUSTAIN
THE MIRACLE OF LIFE.

Claire Small, Body Donor, 1979

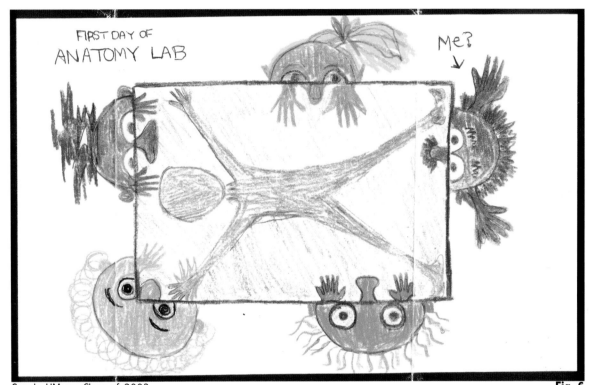

Sarah, UMass, Class of 2003

Fig. 6

3. Meeting the Cadaver

Lectures, films, arts, and poetry are not enough to prepare students for the surrealistic experience of the human anatomy lab. The Inaugural Session always concludes with small-group tours of the dissection laboratory, conducted by Cell Biology faculty and, at times, second-year students, who have already been through the course. This is when the medical students meet the cadavers that they will be dissecting for the whole year. Because UMass draws donors from the surrounding communities, care is taken to ensure, if any student knows of a recent body donor, that that cadaver will not be used by any student in the class.

Actual dissection begins the following day.

4. Later in the Dissection Course: Coping Styles

Usually in October, just before the medical students dissect the head and neck, the course again explores the experience of dissection. The dissection of the head and skull (as well as the hands and genitals) is known to be hard for students — and in some cases traumatic. This session features a compilation of (now former) students' responses to the initial assignment to fill in the blank template and provide a written description. Since 2001, in the darkness and anonymity of the amphitheater, as projected images provide the only light, student voices articulate the range of feelings, fears, and fantasies that their predecessors had written down in their image explanations and that their peers at Weill Medical College had expressed in their journals.

Throughout the year, special lunchtime sessions are scheduled; for example, one session includes the screening and discussion of a film depicting the Netherlands Dance Company's version of Rembrandt's *Anatomy Lesson* (Fig. 7). Often these seminars are triggered by a variety of pertinent recommended readings, the most popular being chapters from Irving Stone's *The Agony and the Ecstasy* (1961), depicting the young artist Michelangelo sneaking into the basement of a monastery so he could learn anatomy for his sculpture and frescoes.

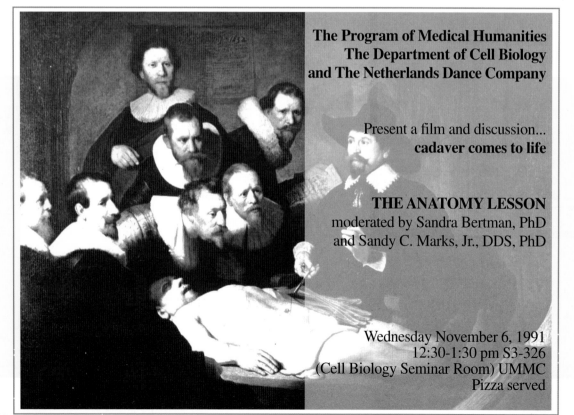

The Program of Medical Humanities
The Department of Cell Biology
and The Netherlands Dance Company

Present a film and discussion...
cadaver comes to life

THE ANATOMY LESSON
moderated by Sandra Bertman, PhD
and Sandy C. Marks, Jr., DDS, PhD

Wednesday November 6, 1991
12:30-1:30 pm S3-326
(Cell Biology Seminar Room) UMMC
Pizza served

Fig. 7

5. Student Service of Thanksgiving for Body Donors

The anatomy course always culminates with a student-designed memorial service in which medical students — through their own rituals, words, and music — pay tribute to the cadavers for the gifts of their bodies.

The family members of the body donors and the entire UMass community are invited to the event, which has mushroomed from a rather small gathering on a school weekday (Fig. 8) to an enormous occasion, moved off campus and held on the weekend to accommodate the large number of guests. The poem on this page, written by a former medical student and read in that year's memorial service, speaks eloquently from the body donor's perspective.

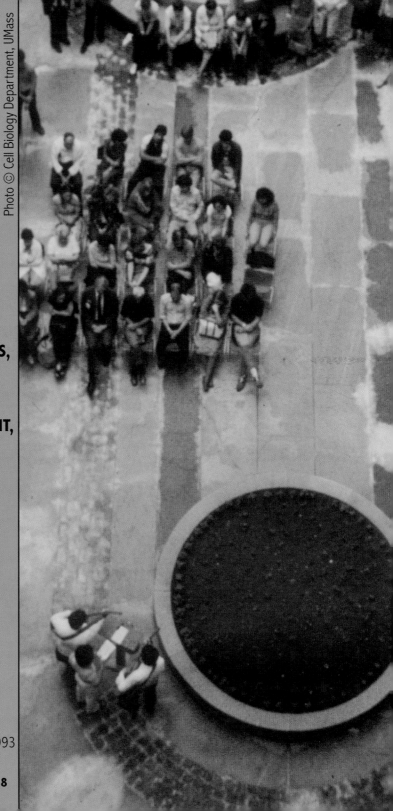

Photo © Cell Biology Department, UMass

IF THE DEAD COULD SPEAK

**IN A WORLD
THAT OFTEN SEEMS ONLY TO TAKE,
WE CHOSE TO GIVE.
WE GAVE NOT OF OUR POSSESSIONS,
BUT OF OURSELVES.**

**THROUGH OUR BLIND EYES,
WE PRAY THAT YOU WILL GAIN SIGHT,
AND THROUGH
OUR WEAKENED MUSCLES,
MAY YOU FIND STRENGTH.**

**ALTHOUGH OUR HEARTS
ARE NOW QUIET
THEY ONCE THUNDERED
WITH THE ÉLAN OF OUR SOULS.
SO WE ASK OF YOU
PLEASE REMEMBER.**

**FOR IT IS THROUGH YOU
THAT OUR END
WILL BRING
NEW BEGINNINGS.**

Kimberly Lonis, UMass, Class of 1993

Fig. 8

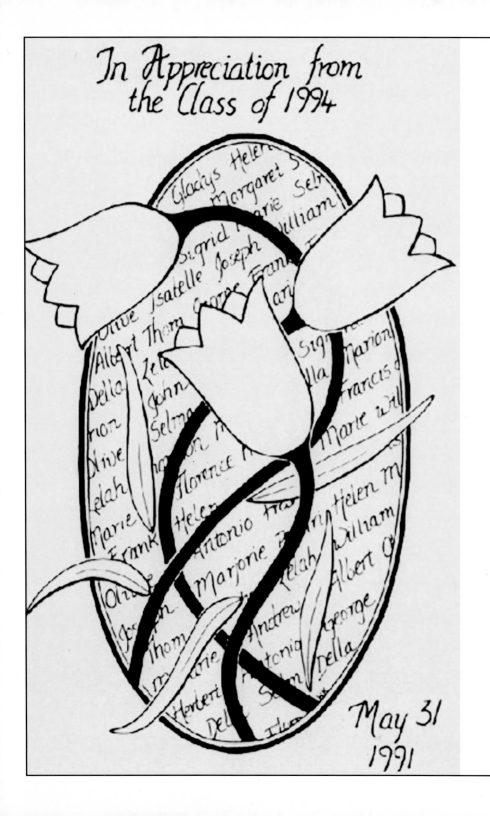

In Appreciation from the Class of 1994

May 31 1991

To the Class of 1994:

We extend our congratulations and best wishes and offer these images you shared with us four years ago.

Thanks for the memories which we will continue to cherish.

John Cooke   *Sandra Betnun*   *Sandy Marks*

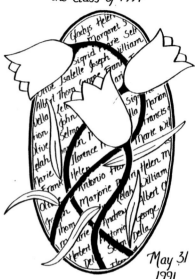

In Appreciation from the Class of 1994

May 31 1991

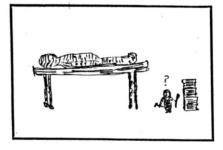

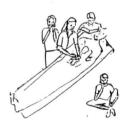

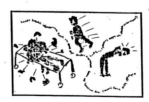

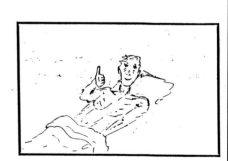

Fig. 9

6. Graduation Tradition

A relatively recent, short-lived tradition was that a few days prior to graduation day, UMass medical graduates — new doctors — received a collection of the images they drew in August of their first year before their anatomy course. Thus they are reminded of their anticipation and the range of emotions expressed before they met and dissected the cadaver — four years earlier(Figs. 9-11). That compilation of memories included the same cover as their thanksgiving service for body donors, reminding them of their first year and how far they have progressed.

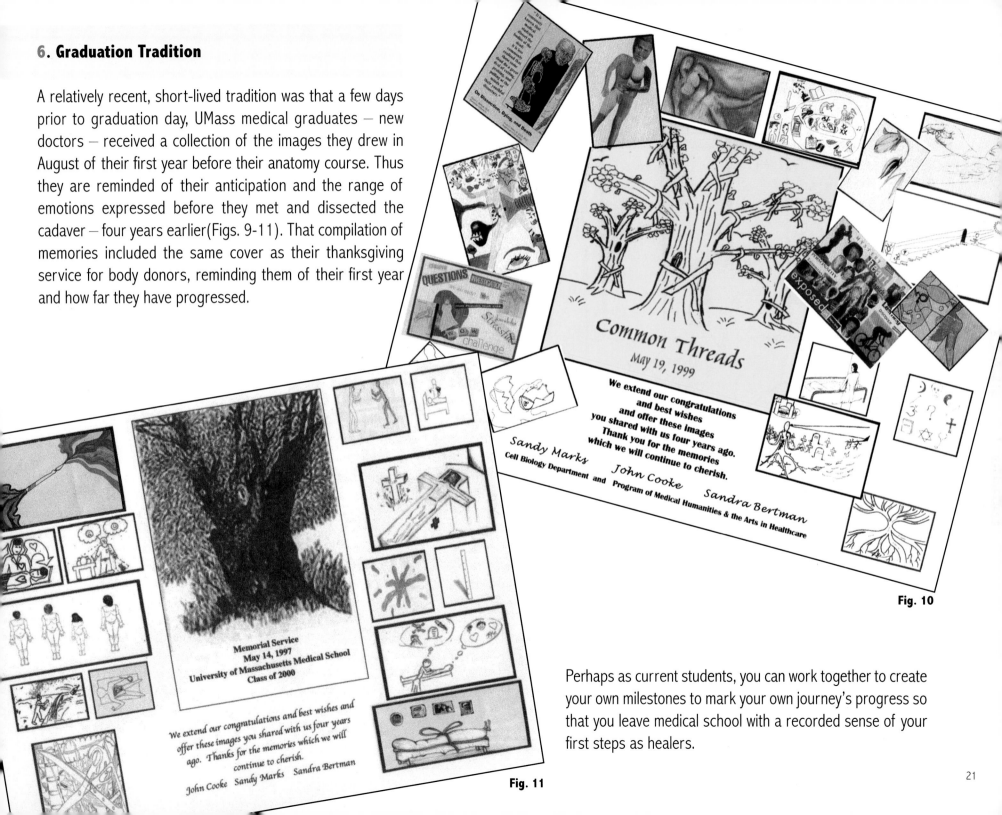

Fig. 10

Fig. 11

Perhaps as current students, you can work together to create your own milestones to mark your own journey's progress so that you leave medical school with a recorded sense of your first steps as healers.

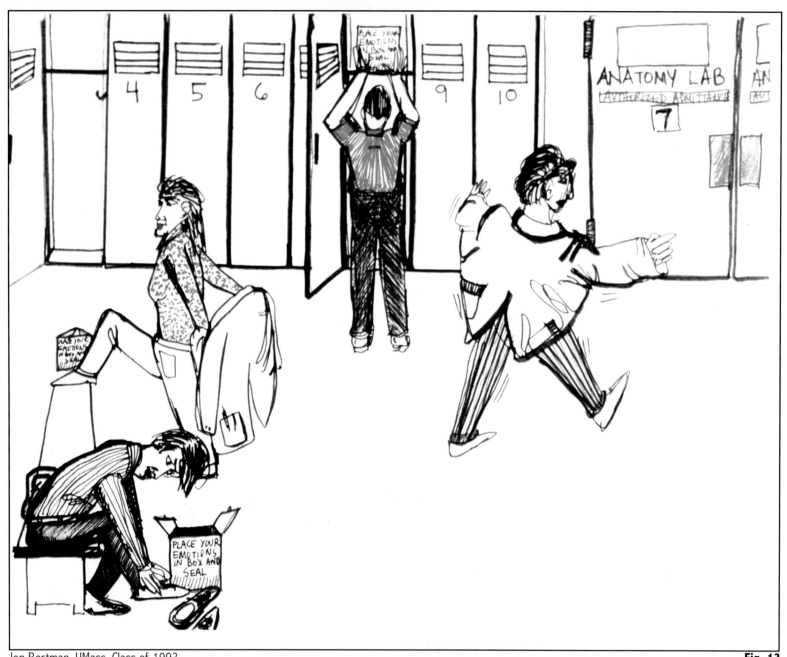

Jon Bertman, UMass, Class of 1993

Fig. 12

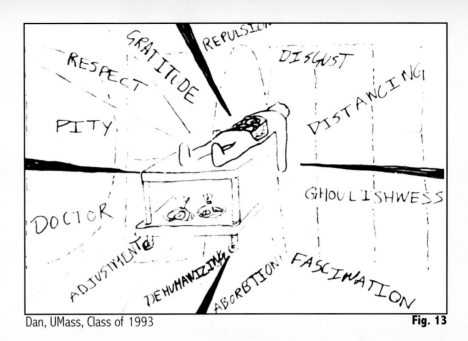

Dan, UMass, Class of 1993   **Fig. 13**

IT IS OUR RESPONSIBILITY TO REMEMBER THAT MEDICINE IS NOT ONLY A SCIENCE, BUT ALSO THE ART OF LETTING OUR OWN INDIVIDUALITY INTERACT WITH THE INDIVIDUALITY OF THE PATIENT.

ALBERT SCHWEITZER, MD, 1968

The Art and Science of Medicine

This publication offers you an opportunity to view former medical students' drawings and thoughts to address your views about dissection, as well as death evoked by the cadaver. If left unattended, these complex feelings and thoughts related to the anatomy experience may impact your later care of patients. In retrospect, many contemporary physicians identify with pediatrician Frances Sharkey (1982) who traced her "emotional detachment" as she made her way through the dissection experience; she often dreamed of her cadaver but says, "I never told this to my fellow students. We didn't talk about the effects our cadavers had on us."

It was then the accepted, even preferred, method to teach medical students to pretend to be detached, to encourage them to act without feelings about the cadaver (Fig.12).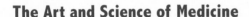

Now more and more medical education centers are seeking creative means of encouraging students to examine their feelings toward dissection. Why didn't Sharkey talk about her dreams of the cadaver, or why didn't her fellow students discuss the effect the cadavers had upon themselves? And what is gained through acknowledging these attitudes and emotions? We hope that you will take some time to discuss these issues with one another and with your faculty.

As students of medicine, you must quickly discover the difficult balance between clinical detachment and feelings of empathy. "The sensitive practitioner knows when to be objective, analytical, and distant. So, too, does she [or he] know when to be confessional, engaged, and intimate." (Benjamin,1984)

Professionalism in medicine requires the acknowledgment of the contradictions that plague us all; in other words, to be an astute practitioner is to possess the complex skill of holding two, or more, opposing truths in balance (Fig. 13). Being able to maintain the creative tension – to see reality in the round – is essential for the healing power of clinicians, the best of whom are able to share their humanity as they practice their science. As Abigail Zuger, MD has written about medical students: "[They] cannot identify too closely with their cadavers, or with their patients in years to come, or they will become paralyzed by emotion." Zuger suggests that even with their "first patient," students must find some kind of a steadiness and self-confidence, somewhere between detached objectivity and emotional involvement.

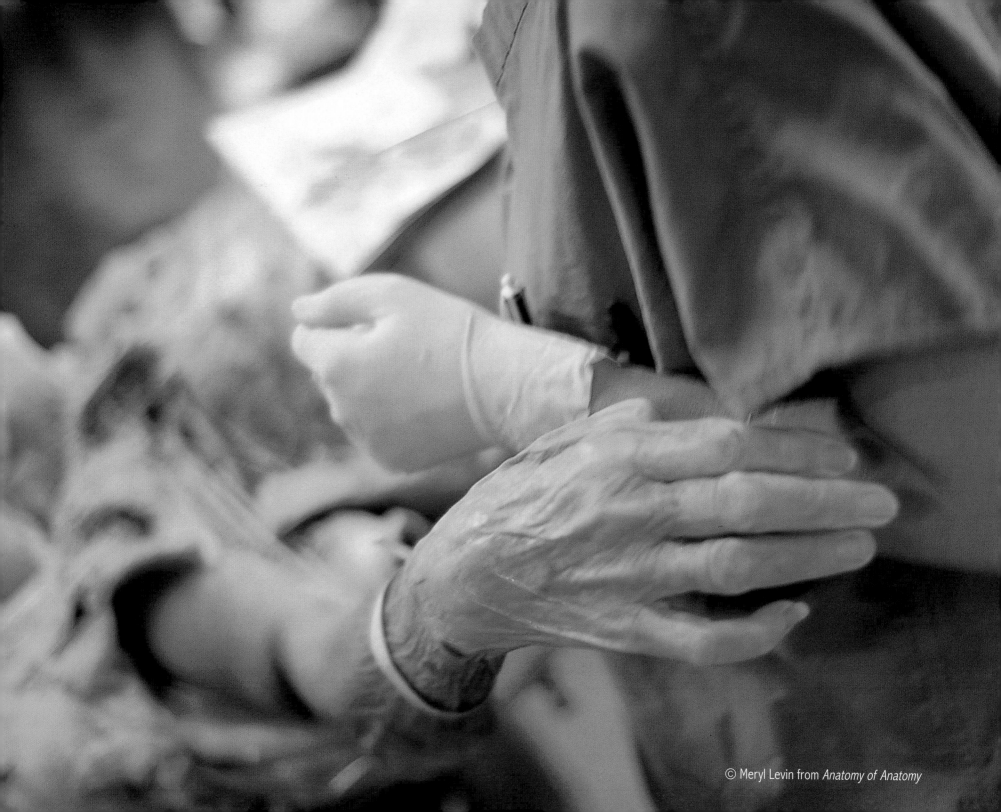

ONE BREATH APART

YOU CAME TO TAKE ME FOR A WALK WITH YOU.
I WAS AFRAID AT FIRST
TO MEET YOU,
TO TAKE YOUR HAND.
I PRETENDED YOU WERE HERE
TO TEACH ME THE DETAILS—
MUSCLES, ARTERIES, NERVES—
AND I HELD ON TIGHT.

THEN I SAW YOUR FACE,
AND I KNEW
YOU CAME TO TAKE ME FOR A WALK WITH YOU—
ON THE EDGE
YOU ON ONE SIDE,
ME ON THE OTHER,
WE ARE ONE BREATH APART.

Nancy Long, UMass, Class of 1995

In the course of acquiring balance and objectivity, students typically review their relationships with their cadavers and acknowledge the cadaver's role as mentor and friend.

The poem on this page, written and read by a medical student at one UMass memorial gathering, admits to fear at the beginning, and describes how the relationship between the student and body donor evolves, by the end of the dissection course, to an enduring memory of gratitude and partnership.

OUR HUMAN FRAME, OUR GUTTED MANSION, OUR ENVELOPING SACK OF BEEF AND ASH IS YET A GLORY.

LEONARD BASKIN, ARTIST, 1963

MEDICAL STUDENTS MEET CADAVERS
MEDICAL STUDENTS FACE DISSECTION

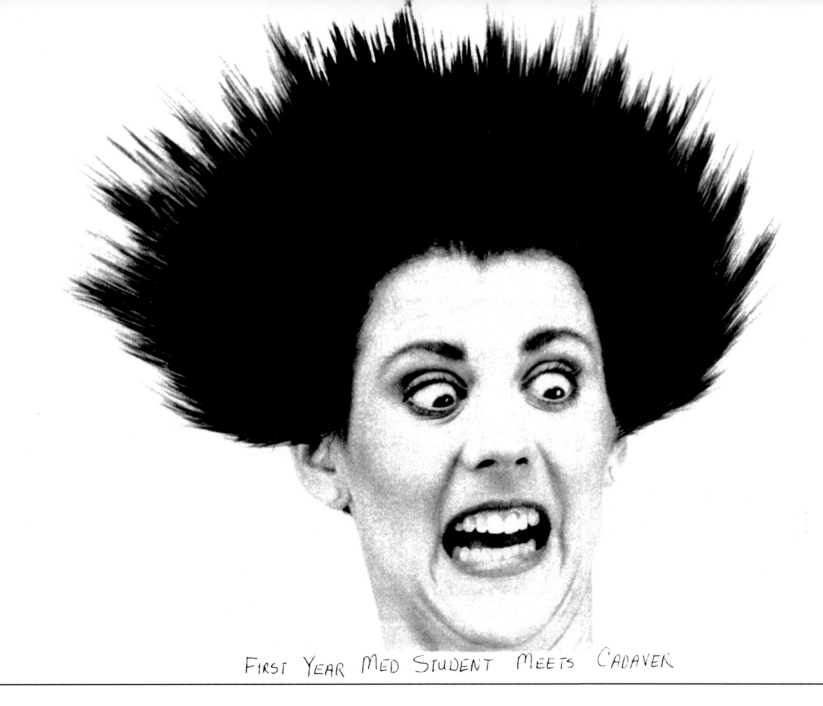

FIRST YEAR MED STUDENT MEETS CADAVER

 But few of us had experienced human anatomy in the way we would during those first months of medical school.

ANATOMY LAB SYMBOLIZES THE MEDICAL STUDENT'S UNOFFICIAL INITIATION INTO MEDICAL SCHOOL. ALL OF US HAVE ABSORBED LECTURES, CONSUMED TEXTBOOKS, AND BATTLED EXAMS. **BUT FEW OF US HAD EXPERIENCED HUMAN ANATOMY IN THE WAY WE WOULD DURING THOSE FIRST MONTHS OF MEDICAL SCHOOL**. I KNOW PEOPLE WHO APPROACHED ANATOMY LAB WITH RELISH. I ALSO KNOW PEOPLE WHO EXPERIENCED APPREHENSION AND A SENSE OF DREAD. **"**

Anonymous, UMass, Class Unknown

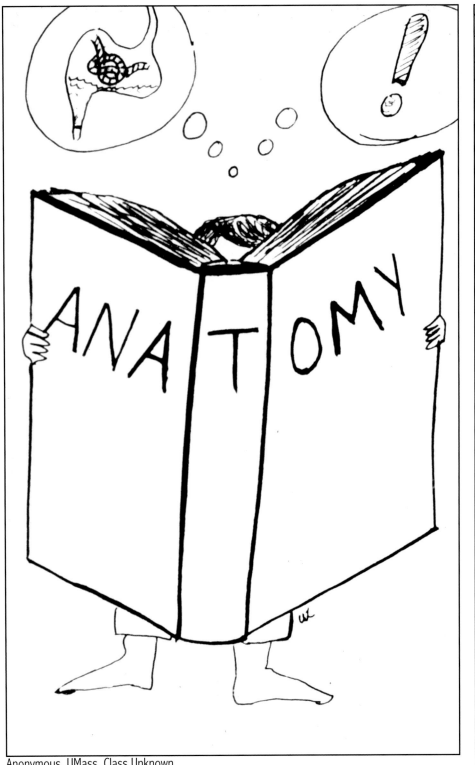

Anonymous, UMass, Class Unknown

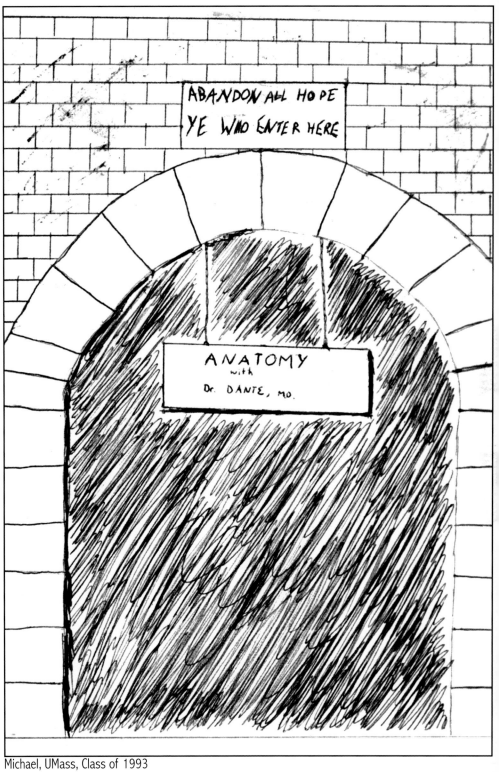

Michael, UMass, Class of 1993

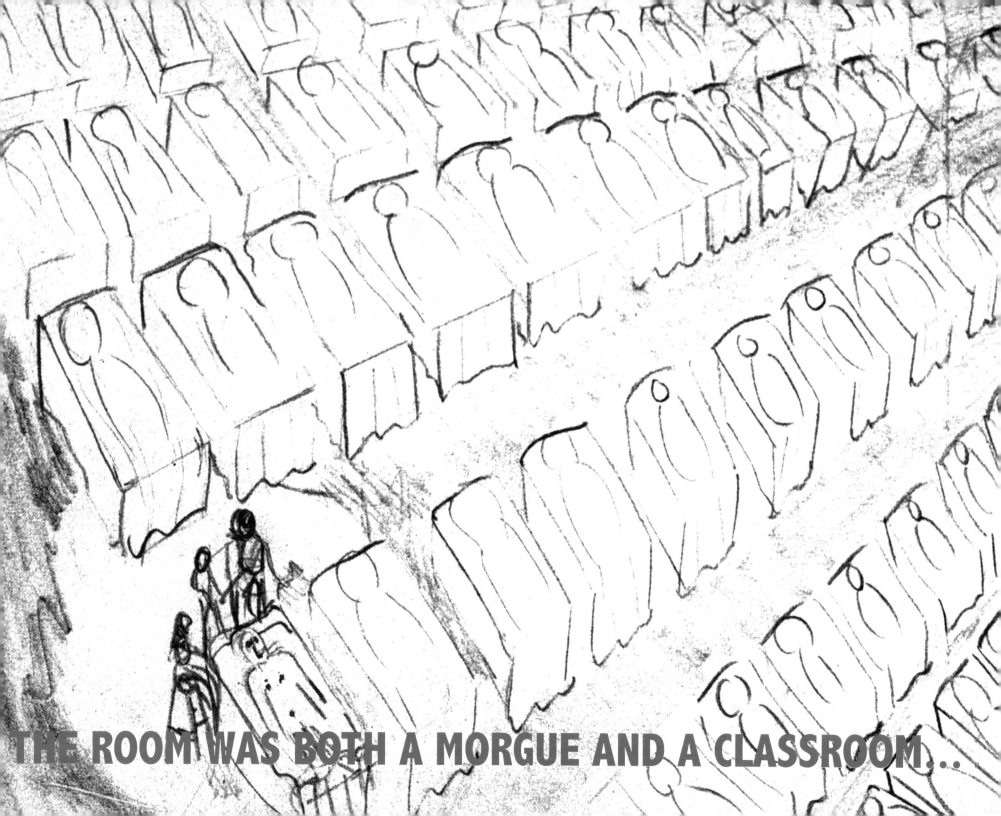

THE ROOM WAS BOTH A MORGUE AND A CLASSROOM...

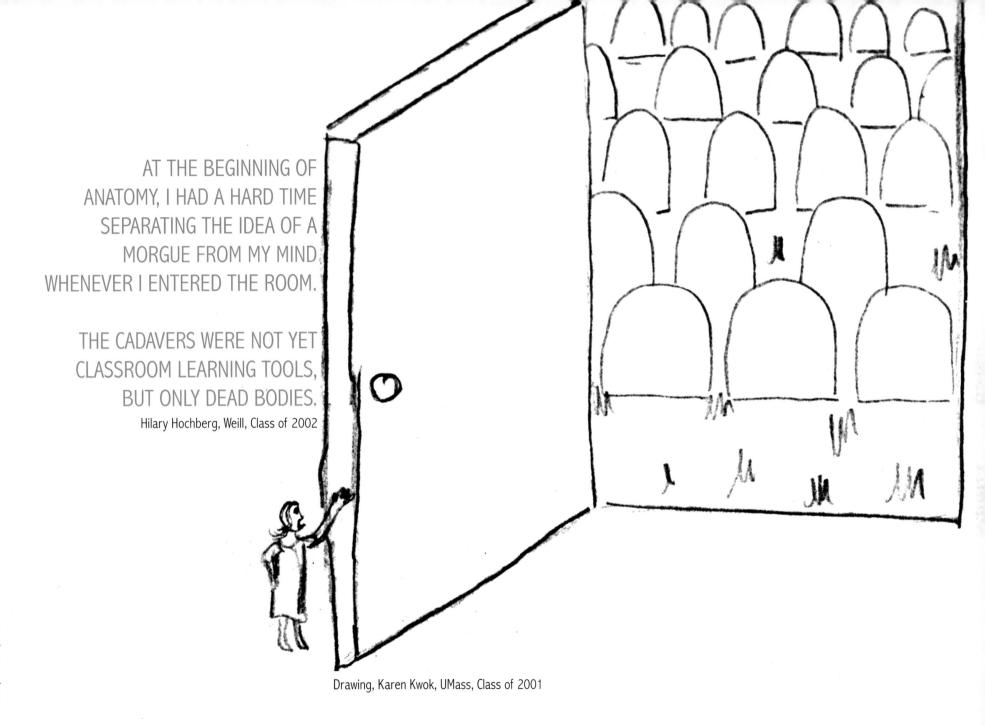

AT THE BEGINNING OF
ANATOMY, I HAD A HARD TIME
SEPARATING THE IDEA OF A
MORGUE FROM MY MIND
WHENEVER I ENTERED THE ROOM.

THE CADAVERS WERE NOT YET
CLASSROOM LEARNING TOOLS,
BUT ONLY DEAD BODIES.

Hilary Hochberg, Weill, Class of 2002

Drawing, Karen Kwok, UMass, Class of 2001

Drawing, Patricia, UMass, Class of 1993

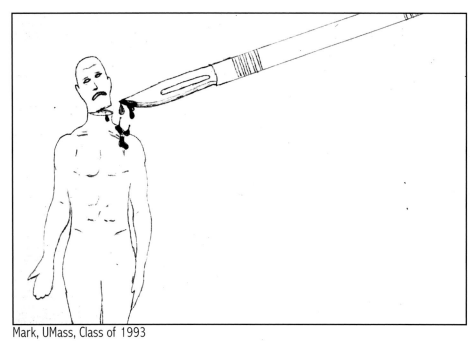

Mark, UMass, Class of 1993

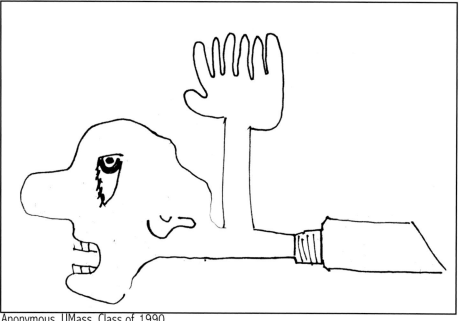

Anonymous, UMass, Class of 1990

I'M MUCH MORE UNCOMFORTABLE HAVING TO DRAW SOMETHING THAN HAVING TO DISSECT SOMEONE.

Anonymous, UMass, Class of 2001

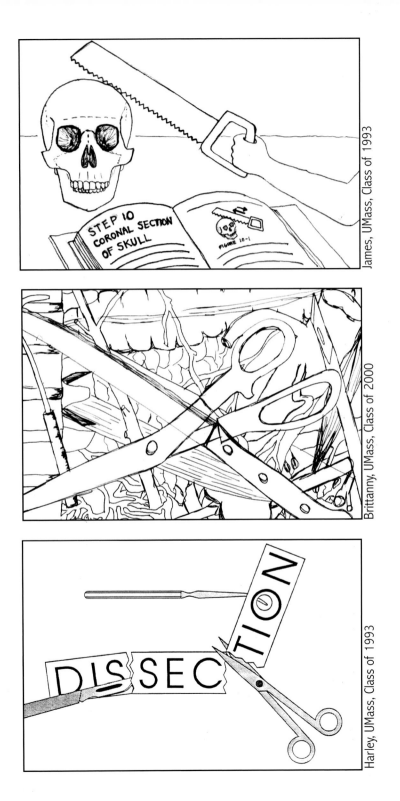

James, UMass, Class of 1993

Brittanny, UMass, Class of 2000

Harley, UMass, Class of 1993

33

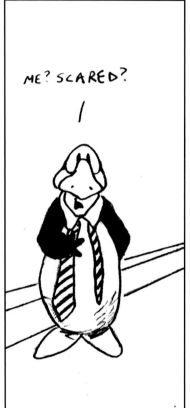
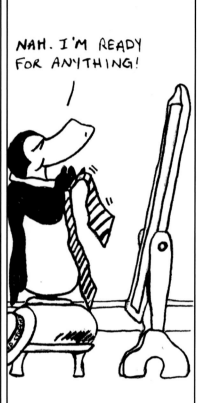
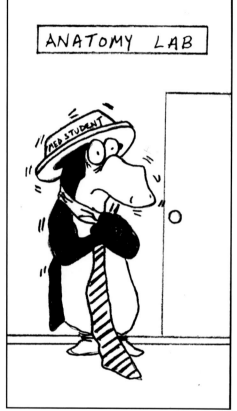

Robert, UMass, Class of 1993

I HAVE BEEN COMPLAINING A LOT. ACTUALLY, IT'S MORE LIKE VOCALIZING MY DISLIKE FOR GROSS ANATOMY.

I HATE IT. I REALLY DO.

I HATE IT.

I HATE IT.

PHEW. IT FEELS GOOD TO WRITE THAT — THERAPEUTIC IN A WAY.

EMOTIONALLY, I'VE BEEN JUMPING ON AND OFF THE BIGGEST, SCARIEST ROLLER COASTER OF MY LIFE.

SOMETIMES I FEEL CONFIDENT, EXCITED, PROFESSIONAL, AND SHALL I DARE TO SAY, SMART?

MOST OF THE TIME, THOUGH, I FEEL VERY SMALL, INSIGNIFICANT, OVERWHELMED, OUT-BATTLED, OUT-SMARTED, OUT-WITTED, AND TOTALLY AND COMPLETELY OUT OF MY LEAGUE.

Carrie Zinamen, Weill, Class of 2002

THE SHEER VOLUME OF MATERIAL AND THE REALITY THAT THE PERSON ON THE TABLE WAS ACTUALLY AT ONE POINT A LIVING, BREATHING SOUL OVERWHELMED ME. I REMEMBER FEELING UNSURE OF MYSELF, MY CONFIDENCE RATTLED TO THE BONE. . . . .

David Hass, Weill, Class of 2002

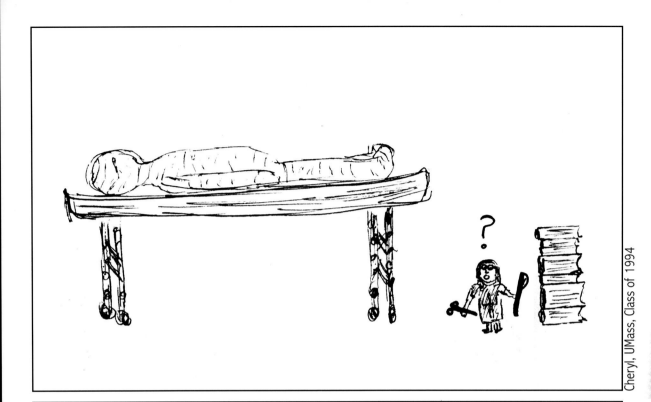

Cheryl, UMass, Class of 1994

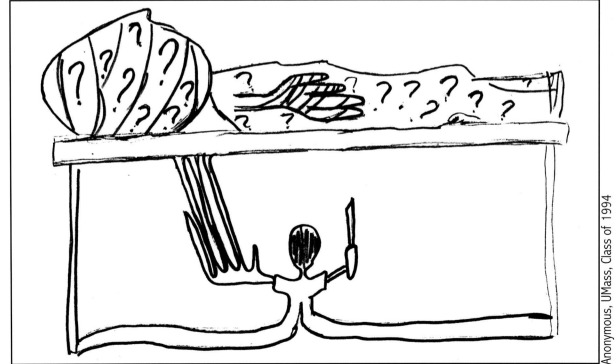

Anonymous, UMass, Class of 1994

IN THE COFFIN LIES THE CADAVER WAITING TO BE USED.
THE SIX INTERACTIONS (FROM TOP LEFT, GOING CLOCKWISE) ARE THE CLOSEST I COME TO UNDERSTANDING MY FEELINGS TOWARD DISSECTION.

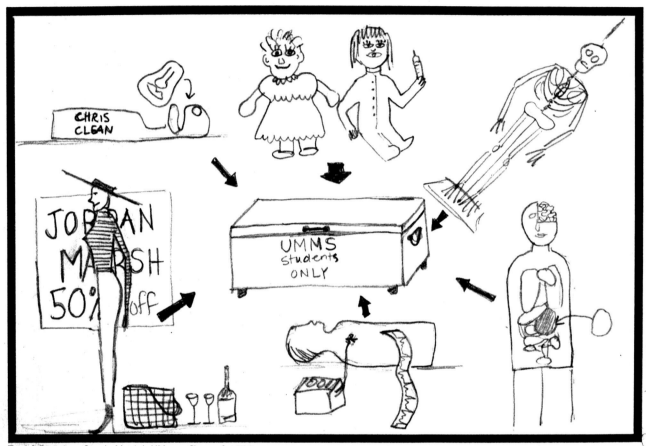

Text & Drawing, Sandy Musial, UMass, Class of 1993

1. CHRIS CLEAN, A DUMMY USED FOR LEARNING CPR
2. DOLLS PLAYED WITH AS A CHILD, THE ONE ON THE RIGHT ABLE TO DRINK AND PEE
3. HANGING SKELETON, USED FOR LEARNING BONES
4. MODEL WITH REMOVABLE ORGANS
5. CPR DUMMY TO PERFECT CPR W/EKG STRIP
6. MANNEQUIN — MADE TO BE HUMAN-LIKE

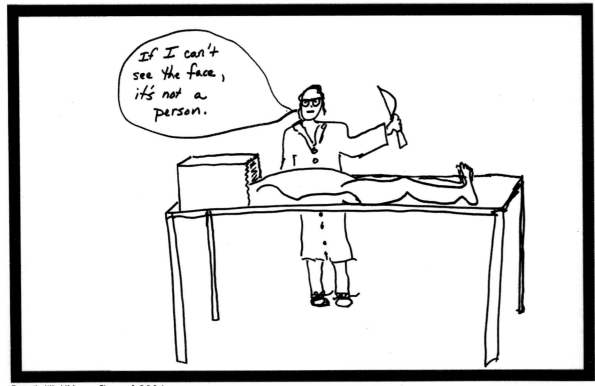

Detail, Jill, UMass, Class of 2004

I DEPICTED MY CADAVER WITHOUT A FACE
BECAUSE I DO NOT SEE HER AS A PERSON.

Anonymous, UMass, Class of 1991

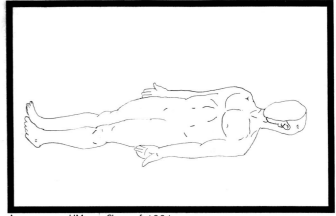

Anonymous, UMass, Class of 1991

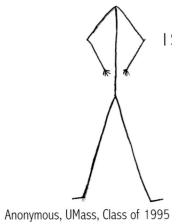

Anonymous, UMass, Class of 1995

I SEE THIS BODY AS A NON-PERSON — AND I PREFER IT THIS WAY.
IS THERE ANYTHING WRONG WITH THIS?

Anonymous, UMass, Class of 1988

I'M JUST AS CONCERNED THAT I WON'T BE BOTHERED
AS I AM ABOUT BEING TOO EMOTIONALLY DISTRAUGHT.

Anonymous, UMass, Class of 2003

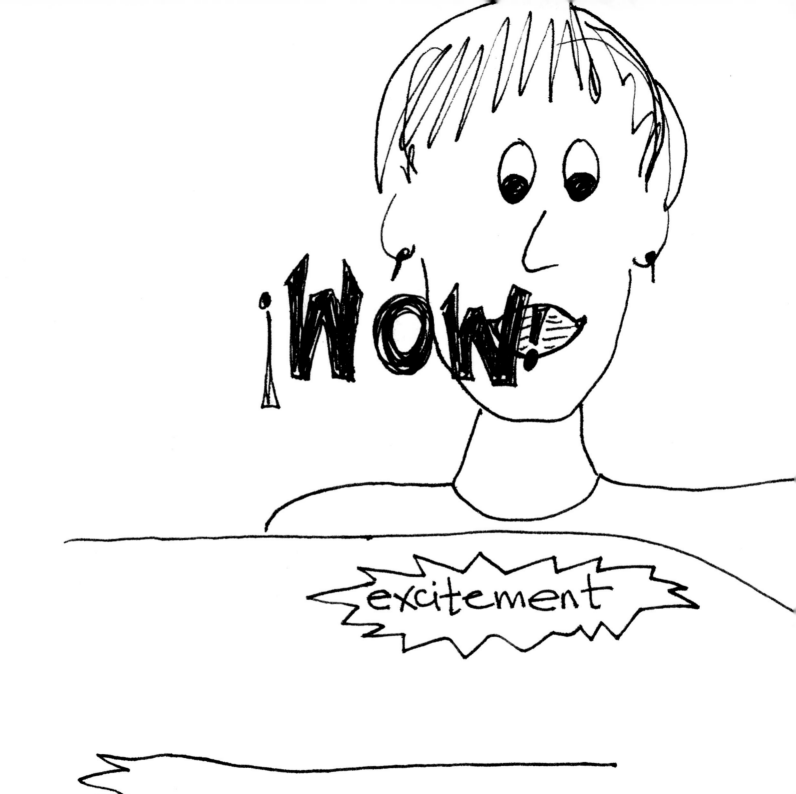

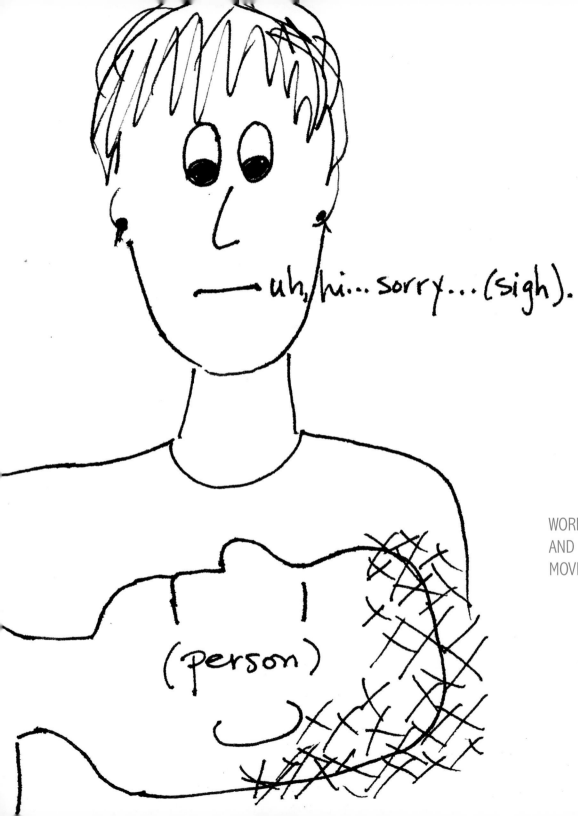

uh, hi... sorry... (sigh).

(person)

WORDS CANNOT DESCRIBE WHAT IT IS LIKE TO PULL BACK A SHEET AND SEE A COLD, ANONYMOUS, VULNERABLE HUMAN BEING — NO MOVEMENT, NO BREATHING, NO SIGNS OF LIFE.

Text, Anonymous, UMass, Class of 1994

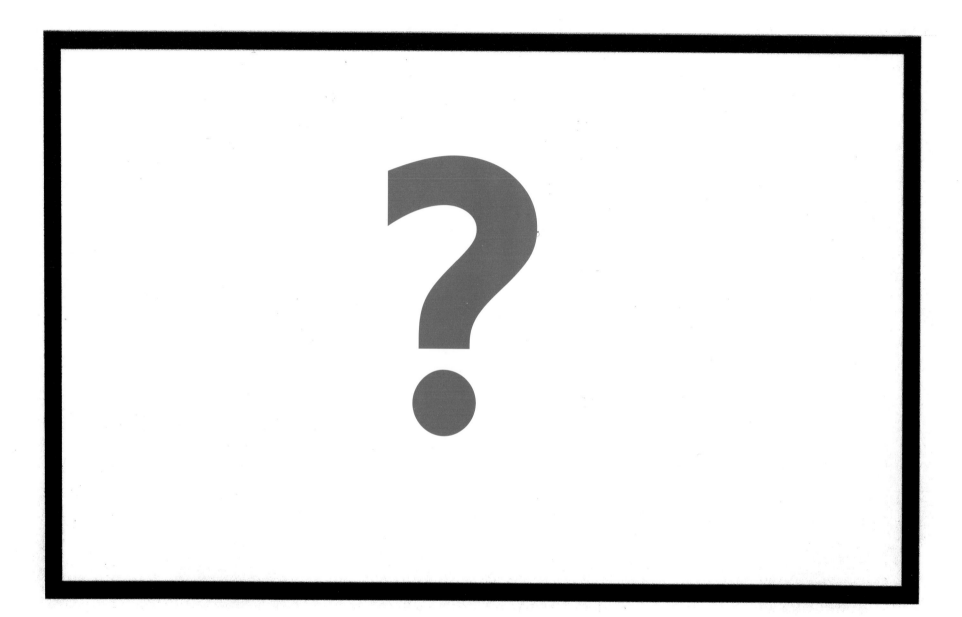

GONE ARE THE LOVERS, THE BURSTS OF LAUGHTER, THE SILENT FEARS, THE SNOWBALL FIGHTS, THE TREES CLIMBED, THE DISLIKE FOR LIMA BEANS, THE PINK SUNRISES, THE FAMILY HUGS AND BASEBALL COLLECTION, THE FAVORITE SONG, THE COMFORT, THE FAITH.

GONE LONG AGO. WHEN THEY LEFT, THEY TOOK IT ALL WITH THEM. HERE NOW THE MAGNIFICENT CLOTHES OF BLOOD AND TENDONS. . . STRONG FRAMES AND ONCE BUSY SYSTEMS COLORED IN BEAUTY — SADLY GRAY NOW THAT THEY HAVE LEFT. . . . ME TOO, SOMEDAY.

Anonymous, UMass, Class of 1994

I HAVE CHOSEN TO LEAVE MY PICTURE BLANK BECAUSE THE THOUGHT OF DISSECTION DOES NOT IMPACT ME. DEATH, I HAVE FOUND, DOES NOT REALLY CONJURE FEELINGS UNLESS IT HAS A PERSONAL CONNECTION FOR ME. A GLANCE AT THE OBITUARIES CAUSE NO EMOTIVE REACTION, UNLESS I HAPPEN ACROSS A NAME I KNOW, THEN THE VOID ONE FEELS IS SIMILAR TO THE BLANK PAGE ALSO.

MANY PEOPLE HAVE HEART ATTACKS, BUT THIS STATEMENT MEANT NOTHING TO ME, UNTIL A PARENT SUFFERED ONE. THE EMOTIONS FELT BY THE "CLOSENESS" OF THIS HEART ATTACK ARE MUCH DIFFERENT WHEN A CONNECTION IS PRESENT. THUS, I WOULD ASSUME THAT MY FEELINGS TOWARDS DISSECTION WILL CHANGE WHEN I SEE AND FEEL THE BODY, BUT, FOR NOW, THE BLANK PAGE IS APPROPRIATE FOR ME.

Michael Kelly, UMass, Class of 2005

THANKS FOR THE EXERCISE. I DIDN'T WANT TO DO IT BUT IT'S BEEN USEFUL.

Anonymous, UMass, Class of 2002

THE BLANK SHEET REPRESENTS THE FACT THAT I HAVEN'T REALLY THOUGHT ABOUT IT. ON THE OTHER HAND, THE CLEAN SPACE IS WAITING TO BE FILLED UP WITH INFORMATION, JUST AS I'M EXCITED TO LEARN ABOUT ANATOMY.

ALSO, THE BLANKNESS HAS NO IDENTITY AS I HOPE THE FACE OF THE CADAVER I WORK ON WILL REMAIN COVERED.

Anonymous, UMass, Class of 2002

LET'S JUST SAY I'M GLAD THERE WAS NO ART SECTION ON THE MCAT.

Anonymous, UMass, Class of 2004

IN SOME WAYS **A BLANK WHITE SHEET** IS THE MOST AUTHENTIC…KNOW NOTHING OF THE PROCESS…NOT EVEN AWARE OF MY FEELINGS.

Anonymous, UMass, Class of 1994

I GREW UP IRISH-CATHOLIC. WE DON'T TALK ABOUT DEATH. WE DON'T TALK ABOUT DYING. AND WE CERTAINLY DON'T TALK ABOUT DISSECTION. IRISH WAKES ARE MERELY AN EXCUSE TO HAVE A FAMILY REUNION. EVERYONE STANDS AROUND CATCHING UP ON OLD TIMES WHILE QUIETLY IGNORING THE "DEARLY DEPARTED," WEARING A CHEAP SUIT AND LIPSTICK, IN THE CORNER. THE PROSPECT OF SEEING THE "BELOVED DEAD" ON A TABLE CONJURES UP ONLY ONE WORD: BIZARRE. MY SCIENTIFIC SELF THINKS DISSECTION WOULD BE AN INCREDIBLE LEARNING EXPERIENCE. HOW OFTEN DOES ONE HAVE THE OPPORTUNITY TO LOOK INSIDE THE HUMAN BODY TO SEE ALL THE GEARS AND NUTS AND BOLTS? BUT MY IRISH-CATHOLIC SELF THINKS DISSECTION IS SOMEWHAT BLASPHEMOUS. WE DON'T EVEN SPEAK ABOUT THE DECEASED, LET ALONE SLICE HIM OPEN. THIS IMAGE REPRESENTS THE TWO WAYS WHICH I PERCEIVE THE BODY WHICH I WILL SOON DISSECT. IT IS A LAYERING OF MY JUXTAPOSED EMOTIONS.

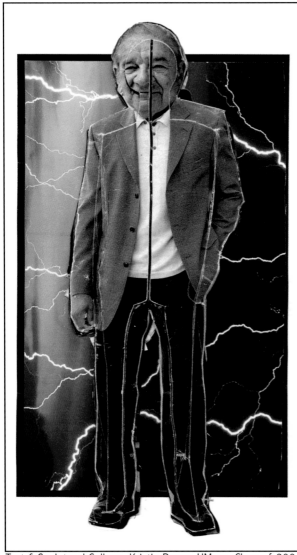 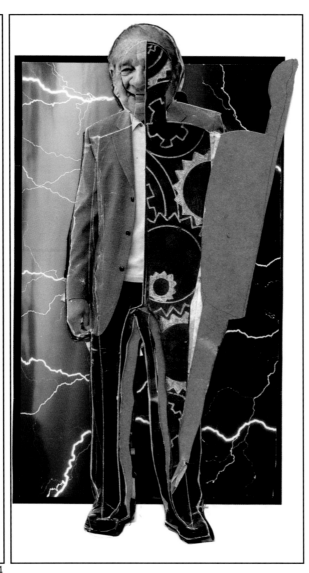 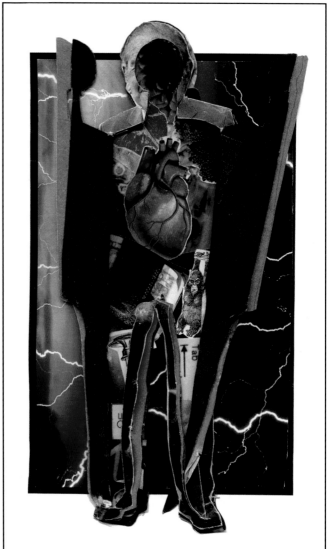

Text & Sculptural Collage, Kristin Burns, UMass, Class of 2004

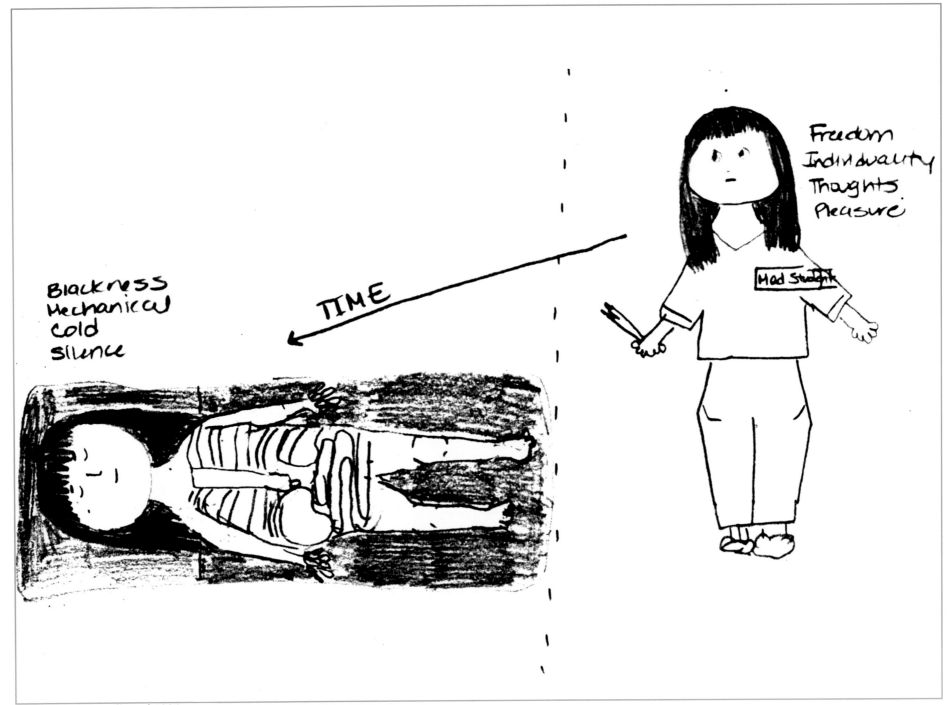

Anonymous, UMass, Class of 1994

IT IS DIFFICULT AT THESE TIMES NOT TO REFLECT UPON THE SIMILARITIES BETWEEN OUR OWN BODIES AND THE COLD CADAVERS BEFORE US. THE HEART THAT WE HOLD IN OUR HANDS ONCE BEAT AS STRONGLY AS THE ONES WITHIN US. THE VESSELS, NOW DRY AND COLLAPSED, ARE SHADOWS OF THE BUSTLING HIGHWAYS OF BLOOD FLOWING TO THE TIPS OF OUR OWN FINGERS. WE LIE IN BED AND FEEL OUR OWN HEARTS PULSING WITHIN OUR OWN BELLIES. AFTER TOUCHING THE SPONGY LUNG, WHICH REBOUNDS WITH EASE AFTER A GENTLE SQUEEZE, WE DRAW DEEP BREATHS AND PICTURE THE DRAMATIC EXPANSION AND CONTRACTION WITHIN OUR OWN CHEST WALLS. . . .

IN A WAY, I WAS REPULSED. I LOOKED AT MY NAKED BODY IN THE SHOWER AND THOUGHT OF HERS. ADMITTEDLY, HER AGED LIFELESS BODY DID NOT HOLD A CLOSE RESEMBLANCE TO MY OWN, BUT I COULDN'T HELP BUT THINK THAT THE LIFE-GIVING BLOOD THAT COURSED THROUGH MY VESSELS WOULD BE TRANSIENT AND SOME DAY STOP; AND I WOULD BECOME LIKE HER. THIS CAUSED ME TO VIEW MY OWN BODY IN A DIFFERENT LIGHT.

Hilary Hochberg, Weill, Class of 2002

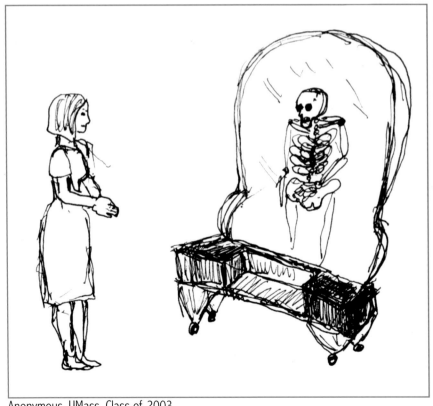

Anonymous, UMass, Class of 2003

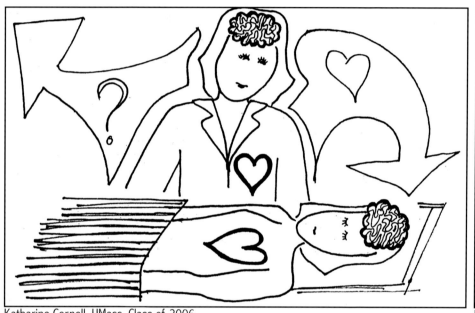

Katharine Cornell, UMass, Class of 2006

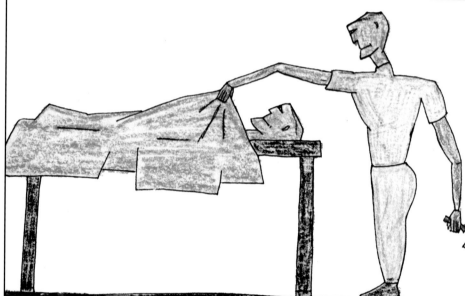

John, UMass, Class of 2006

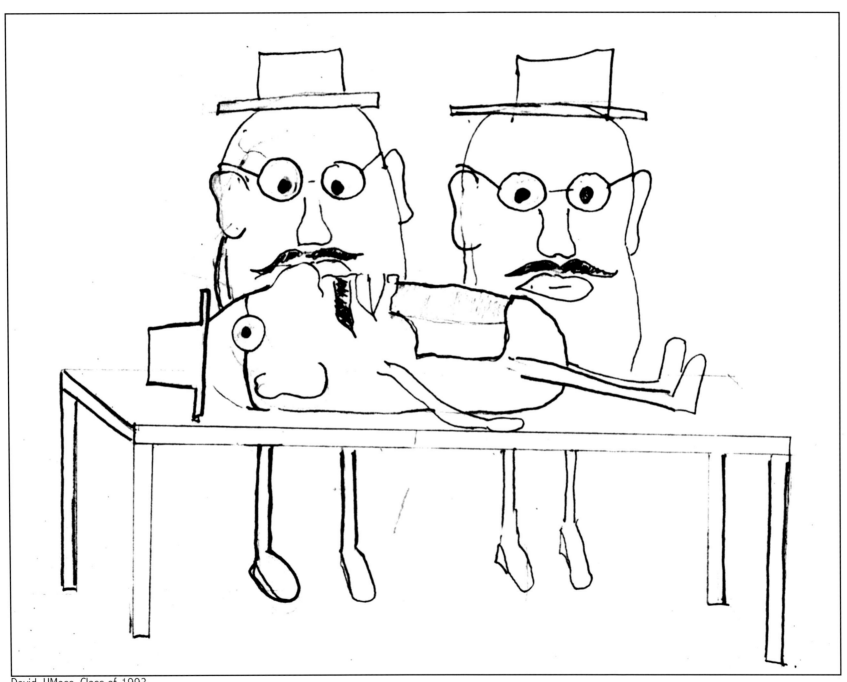

David, UMass, Class of 1993

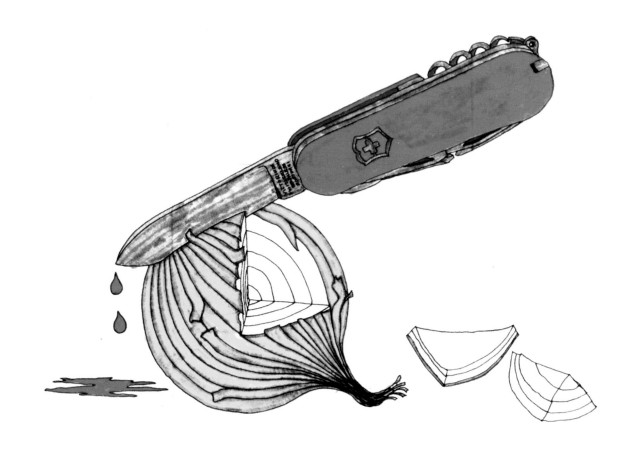

I DREW A SWISS ARMY KNIFE, DRIPPING BLOOD, WHILE CUTTING A YELLOW ONION. THE ONION SYMBOLIZES THE HUMAN BODY. THE YELLOW PEEL REPRESENTS THE FEAR THAT I EXPECT TO FEEL WHEN I FIRST ENCOUNTER A HUMAN CADAVER. THIS ISN'T A FEAR OF DEATH OR EVEN BECOMING SICK, BUT MERELY A FEAR OF THE UNKNOWN: HOW WILL I REACT? WHAT WILL I DO? WILL I FAIL THIS BASIC TEST?

THE WHITE INSIDE OF THE ONION REPRESENTS THE PURITY OF THE KNOWLEDGE THAT I HOPE TO GAIN FROM THE CADAVER. YET, THIS KNOWLEDGE WON'T COME ALL AT ONCE; THE PROCESS OF PEELING THE LAYERS AWAY WILL TAKE TIME.

THE SMELL OF THE ONION REPRESENTS TWO THINGS. FIRST, CADAVERS STINK AND THIS STRONG SMELL PROBABLY BROUGHT THE ONION METAPHOR TO MIND. SECOND, THE SMELL OF THE ONION MAKES SOME PEOPLE CRY. THIS THREAT OF CRYING ALSO EXPRESSES THE FEAR OF THE UNKNOWN THAT I DESCRIBED ABOVE.

I CHOSE A SWISS ARMY KNIFE AS MY CUTTING INSTRUMENT BECAUSE I SEE IT AS A CRUDE YET PRACTICAL BLADE. I FEEL THAT MY FIRST ATTEMPTS AT CUTTING INTO THE HUMAN BODY WILL BE CLUMSY AND UNREFINED BECAUSE OF MY IGNORANCE AND LACK OF PRACTICE.

THE DROPS AND PUDDLE OF BLOOD WERE ADDED AS AN AFTERTHOUGHT. I WAS TRYING TO FIND A SYMBOLIC WAY TO SUGGEST THE HONOR THAT I FEEL FOR THE PERSON WHO SACRIFICED HIS/HER BODY FOR MY EDUCATION. SINCE SPILLING BLOOD HAS BEEN CONSIDERED HONORABLE (I DON'T AGREE, BUT I COULDN'T FIND A BETTER VISUAL WAY TO REPRESENT HONOR AND SACRIFICE), IT SEEMED LIKE THE BEST WAY TO INCORPORATE THAT FEELING. . . .

Text & Drawing, Ian Bach, UMass, Class of 1995

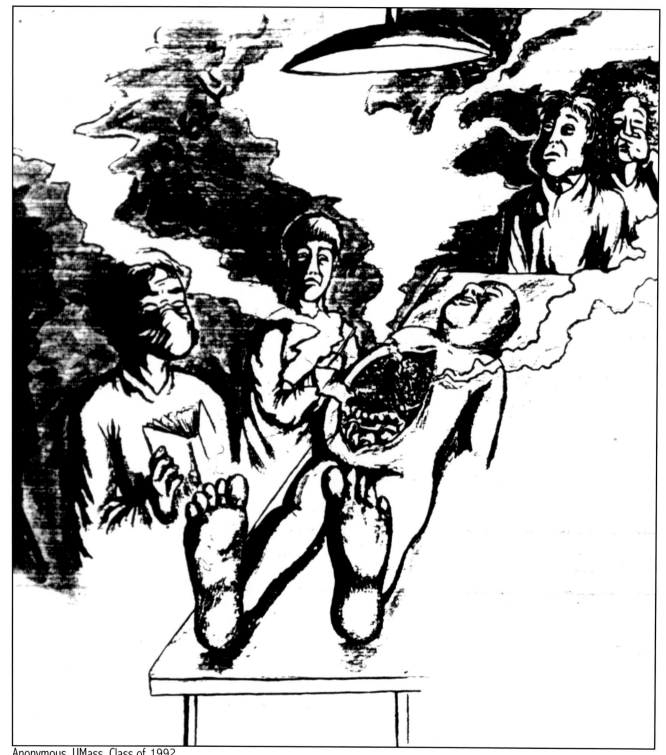

Anonymous, UMass, Class of 1992

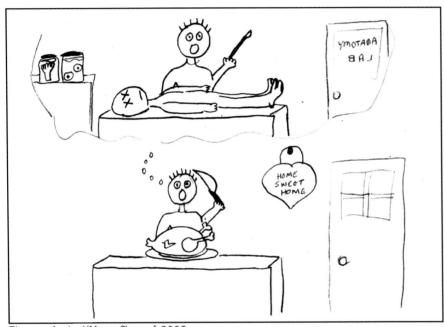

Theresa Arpin, UMass, Class of 2002

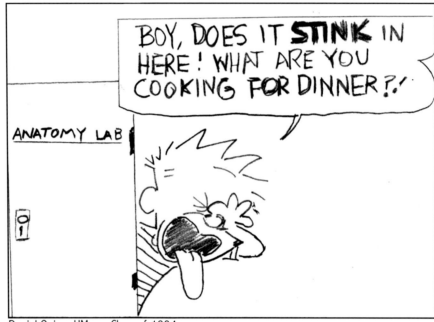

Daniel Quinn, UMass, Class of 1994

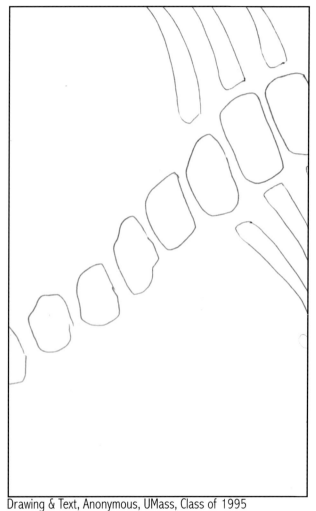

Drawing & Text, Anonymous, UMass, Class of 1995

I KEPT THINKING OF THIS IMAGE, EVEN THOUGH IT DOESN'T SEEM GORY ENOUGH. PROBABLY IT MEANS AT LEAST THE FOLLOWING:

— THAT I IMAGINE AN UNDERLYING ORDER AND BEAUTY THAT WILL BE REVEALED TO ME

— THAT I WILL "GET DOWN TO THE BONES" OR "TO THE HEART OF THINGS" CHOOSING THE RIB CAGE. ALSO, BONES MIGHT SYMBOLIZE DEATH

— THE IMAGE IS ROUGHLY CROSS-SHAPED OR A VERY PECULIAR CROSS.

I AM A CHRISTIAN AND THINK THAT MY FAITH WILL HELP ME HANDLE THE DIFFICULTIES OF BECOMING A DOCTOR INCLUDING CUTTING INTO A HUMAN CORPSE.

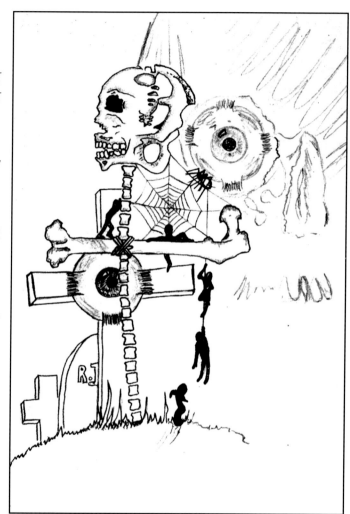

Anonymous, UMass, Class of 1994

SYMBOLISM OF WHAT I ASSOCIATE WITH DEATH AND SACRIFICE: I PICTURE MY CADAVER BEING IN THAT POSITION AS HE LIES ON THE DISSECTION TABLE. I EXTENDED THE CROSS TO THAT OF THE RED CROSS, AN ORGANIZATION AND SYMBOL WE ASSOCIATE WITH SAVING LIVES. BY USING THE CROSS I HAVE LINKED DEATH TO LIFE.

Anonymous, UMass, Class of 1994

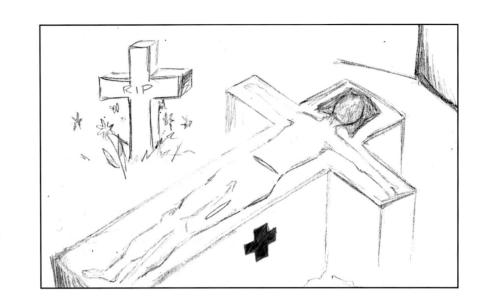

I AM NOT SURE WHETHER I BELIEVE THE SOUL DEPARTS AS SOON AS DEATH OCCURS, OR THAT THE SPIRIT CANNOT BE SET FREE UNTIL THE BODY IS PEACEFULLY LAID TO REST. . . . FOR THE RECORD, I AM NOT A PARTICULARLY RELIGIOUS PERSON.

Stephen, UMass, Class of 1996

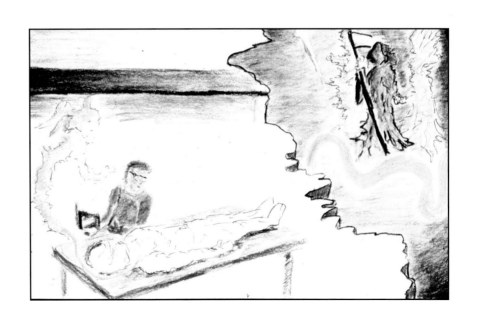

I LIKE THE BUDDHIST NOTION OF DEATH AND THE BODY.
WHEN YOU BREAK A CUP OF TEA, THE TEA SPILLS OUT BUT IT'S
STILL TEA. THE CUP REPRESENTS THE BODY — WHILE STILL A CUP,
IT'S NOW BROKEN. I PUT THE SYMBOLS FOR YIN AND YANG AS
WELL AS INFINITY BECAUSE I ANTICIPATE BEING MARVELED BY HOW
WELL THE BODY IS DESIGNED: THERE IS BALANCE IN
FUNCTION/PHYSIOLOGY AND HARMONY.
ALSO, THERE IS AN INFINITE AMOUNT TO BE LEARNED.
I DO NOT BELIEVE SCIENCE WILL EVER FULLY UNDERSTAND ALL
THAT A HUMAN BODY IS.

Text & Drawing, Matthias, UMass, Class of 2002

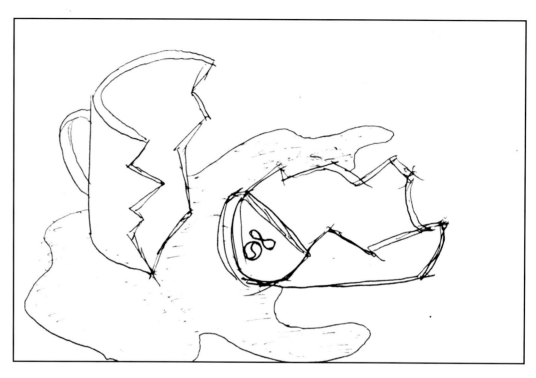

A CANDLE SUGGESTS LIFE GIVING CONTRAST TO THE PEBBLES BELOW.
THE HUMAN BODY IN THE CENTER SIGNIFIES THE FOCUS OF THE CONFLICT:
THE BALANCE BETWEEN OPPOSITES,
BEAUTY/REPULSION,
LOSS OF PERSON/THE DIGNITY OF DONATING ONES BODY.

Text and Drawing, Anonymous, UMass, Class of 1991

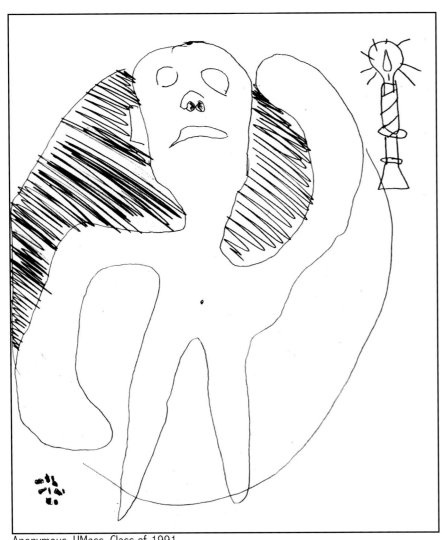

Anonymous, UMass, Class of 1991

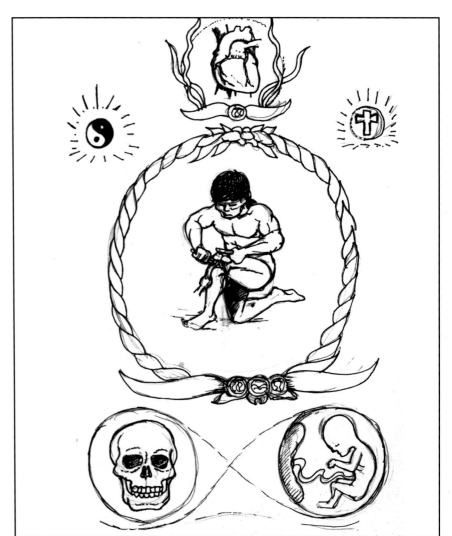

Stephen, UMass, Class of 1993

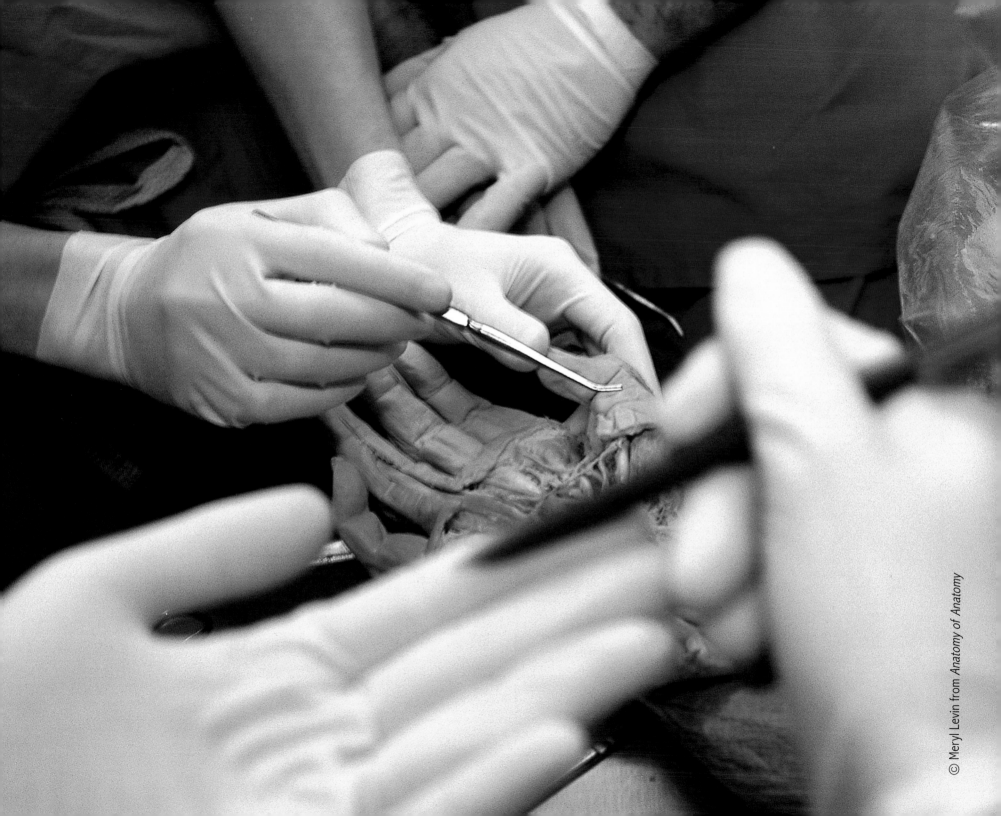

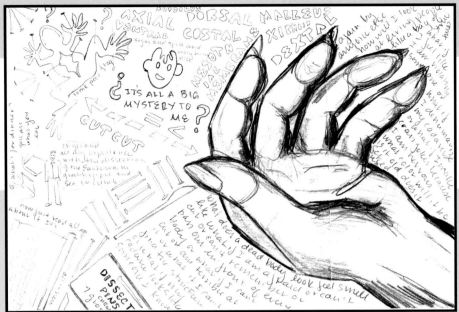

Thad, UMass, Class of 1995

BUT THE HAND HOLDS SO MUCH MORE.
PALM SIDE UP, ITS LINES REVEAL A LIFETIME OF HARD WORK, TENDER TOUCHES, AND EXPLORATION – A LIFETIME NOW COMPLETE.

HOWEVER, THIS HAND WILL CONTINUE TO GIVE.

Anonymous, UMass, Class of 1995

I AM REACHING OUT TO MY CADAVER'S HAND
SHOWING THAT I AM INTERESTED IN THE LIFE HE OR SHE LIVED,
AND SO THANKFUL FOR THE SACRIFICE.

Drawing & Text, Julie, UMass, Class of 2005

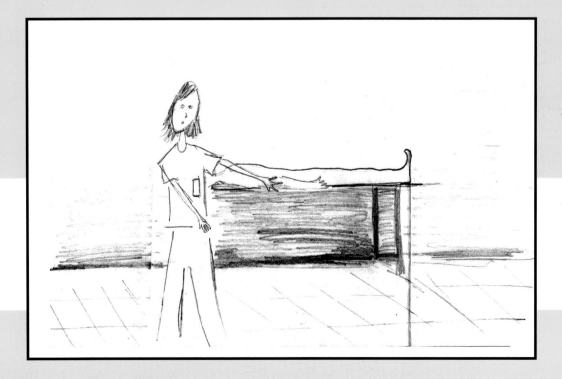

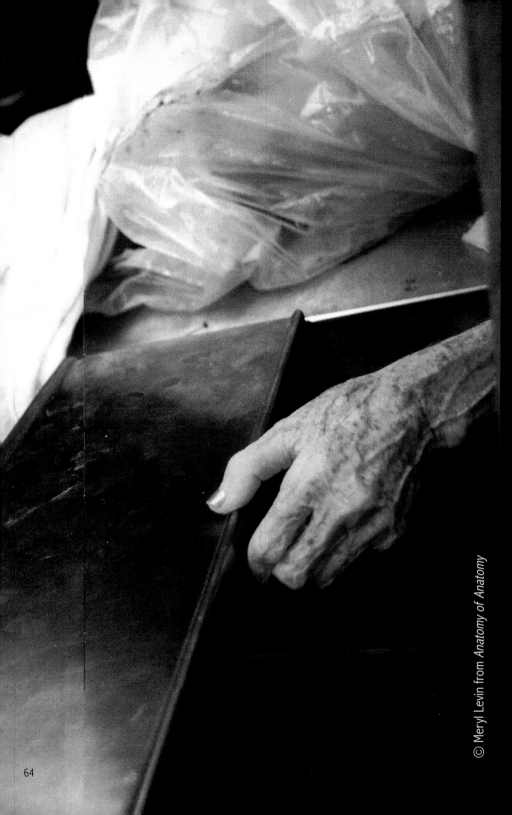

I DIDN'T EXPECT THE BODIES TO BE WEARING FINGERNAIL POLISH, OR HAVE WELL-MANICURED NAILS. THIS ELDERLY BODY HAD ON OPAQUE, WHITISH POLISH WITH BLUE HUES, A COLOR I COULDN'T IMAGINE ON MY OWN GRANDMOTHER. IT WAS FROM THE COLLECTION. . .THAT HAD PERVADED THE FASHION SCENE LAST YEAR, AND THUS FOUND ITS WAY TO THE FINGERS OF MANY SEVENTH GRADE GIRLS. HERE IT WAS ON *HER* NAILS, PERHAPS PAINTED BY HER GRANDDAUGHTER VISITING HER IN THE HOSPITAL. . . .

Hilary Hochberg, Weill, Class of 2002

© Meryl Levin from *Anatomy of Anatomy*

SHE LOOKED SO SMALL, FRAIL, SEXLESS EVEN. BUT THEN I SAW A BLISTER ON HER TOE. AND ON ANOTHER CADAVER, NAIL POLISH. SO THEY WERE HUMAN, ONCE.

Carrie Zinamen, Weill, Class of 2002

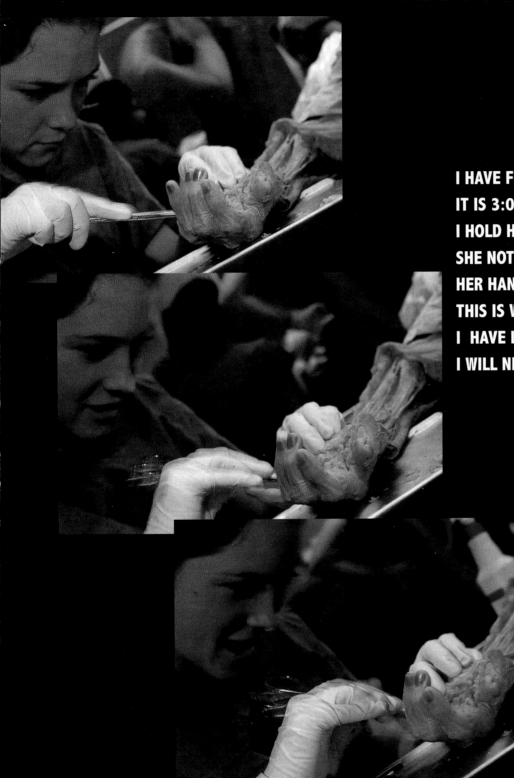

I HAVE FINISHED MY DISSECTION OF THE WRIST AND HAND.

IT IS 3:00 PM, AND I HAVE TO PICK UP MY DAUGHTER FROM SCHOOL.

I HOLD HER HAND TIGHTLY AS WE CROSS THE STREET.

SHE NOTICES, BUT DOESN'T SAY ANYTHING.

HER HAND IS SOFT AND WARM DESPITE THE JANUARY COLD.

THIS IS WHAT LIFE FEELS LIKE, I SAY TO MYSELF.

I HAVE LEARNED SOMETHING ABOUT THE HUMAN TOUCH.

I WILL NEVER HOLD SOMEONE'S HAND THE SAME OLD, IGNORANT WAY AGAIN.

Rajiv Gupta, Weill, Class of 2002

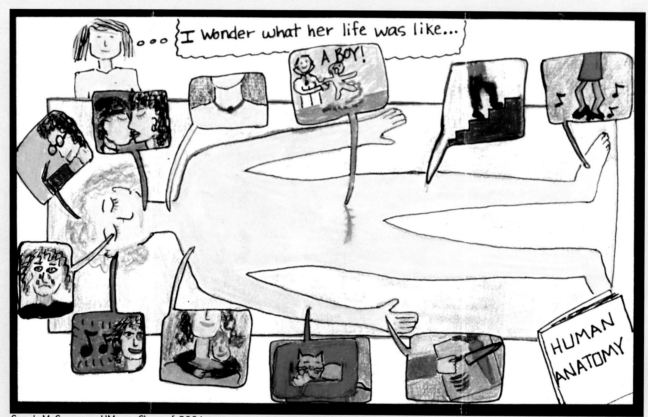

Sarah McSweeney, UMass, Class of 2001

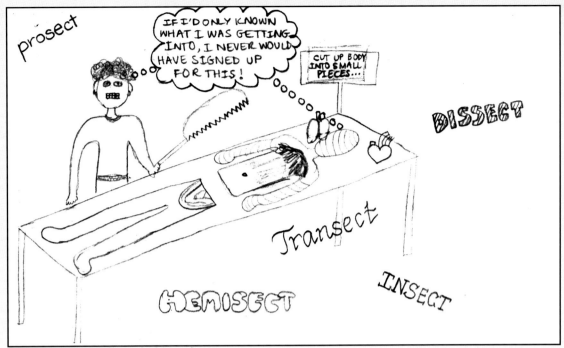

Anonymous, UMass, Class of 1994

I WONDERED WHY SHE DECIDED TO DONATE HER BODY TO SCIENCE, AND THEN I WONDERED IF I COULD MAKE THAT SAME DECISION.

DID SHE KNOW WHAT WAS IN STORE FOR HER WHEN SHE SIGNED THE CONSENT FORM? AS I LOOKED AT ALL THE BLADES AND SCISSORS AND SHARP METAL UTENSILS STREWN AROUND THE ROOM, I WONDERED IF I KNEW WHAT WAS IN STORE FOR THE BOTH OF US.

Hilary Hochberg, Weill, Class of 2002

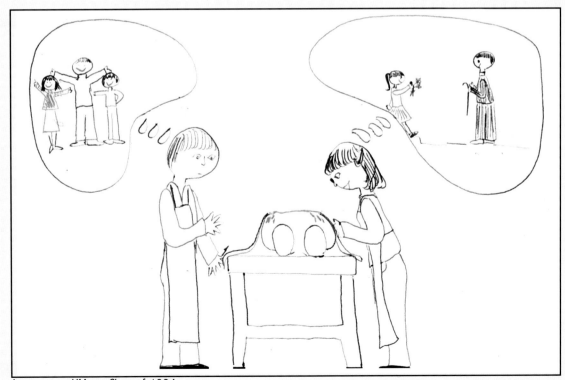

Anonymous, UMass, Class of 1994

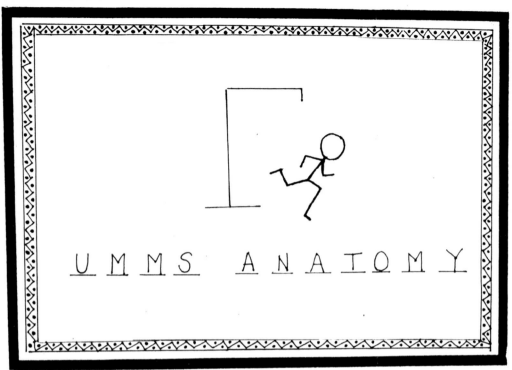

Anonymous, UMass, Class of 2002

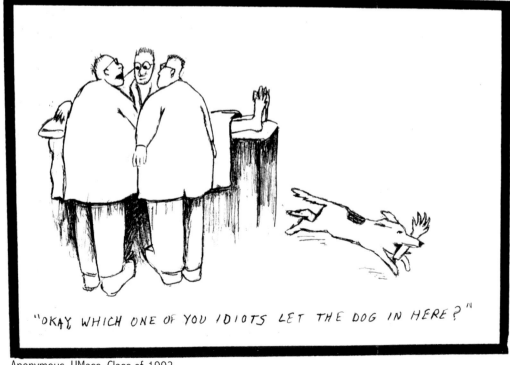

Anonymous, UMass, Class of 1993

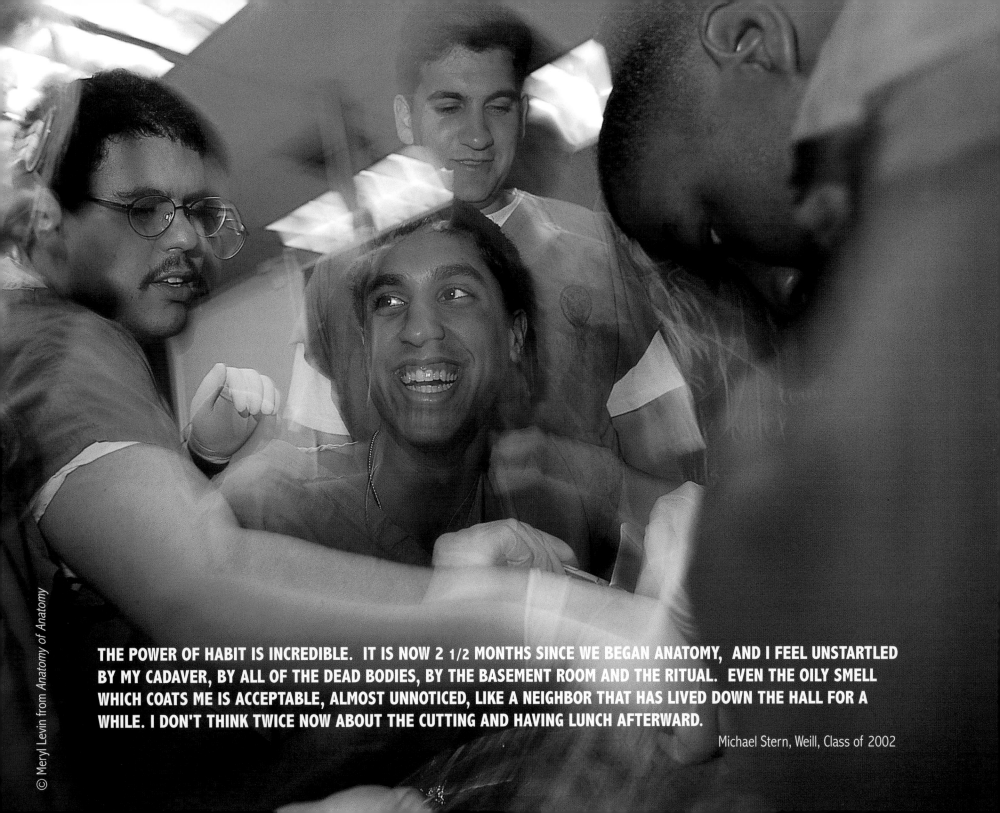

THE POWER OF HABIT IS INCREDIBLE. IT IS NOW 2 1/2 MONTHS SINCE WE BEGAN ANATOMY, AND I FEEL UNSTARTLED BY MY CADAVER, BY ALL OF THE DEAD BODIES, BY THE BASEMENT ROOM AND THE RITUAL. EVEN THE OILY SMELL WHICH COATS ME IS ACCEPTABLE, ALMOST UNNOTICED, LIKE A NEIGHBOR THAT HAS LIVED DOWN THE HALL FOR A WHILE. I DON'T THINK TWICE NOW ABOUT THE CUTTING AND HAVING LUNCH AFTERWARD.

Michael Stern, Weill, Class of 2002

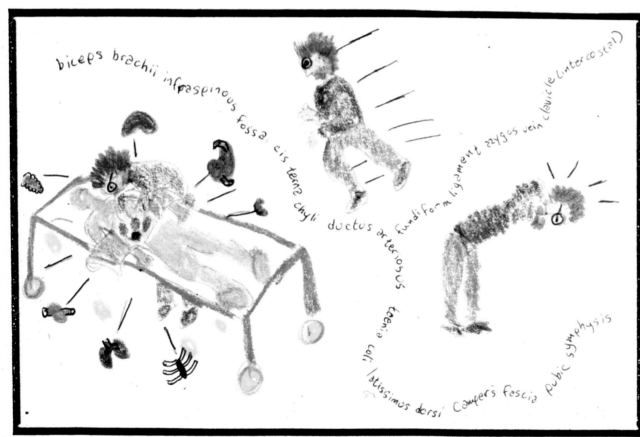

biceps brachii infraspinous fossa eis tenia chyli ductus arteriosus fundiform ligament azygos vein clavicle (intercostal) teenia coli latissimus dorsi Camper's fascia pubic symphysis

Lloyd, UMass, Class of 1994

70

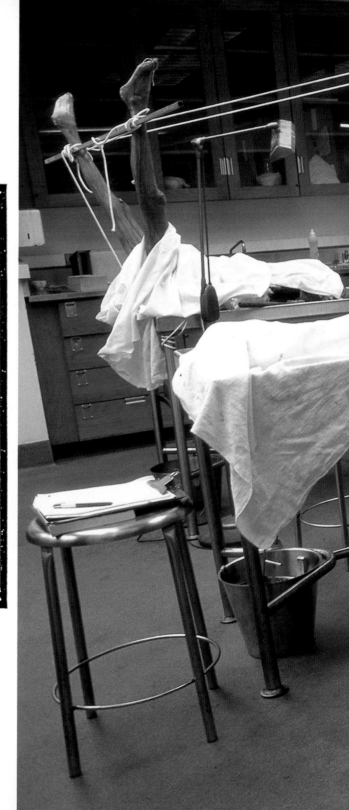

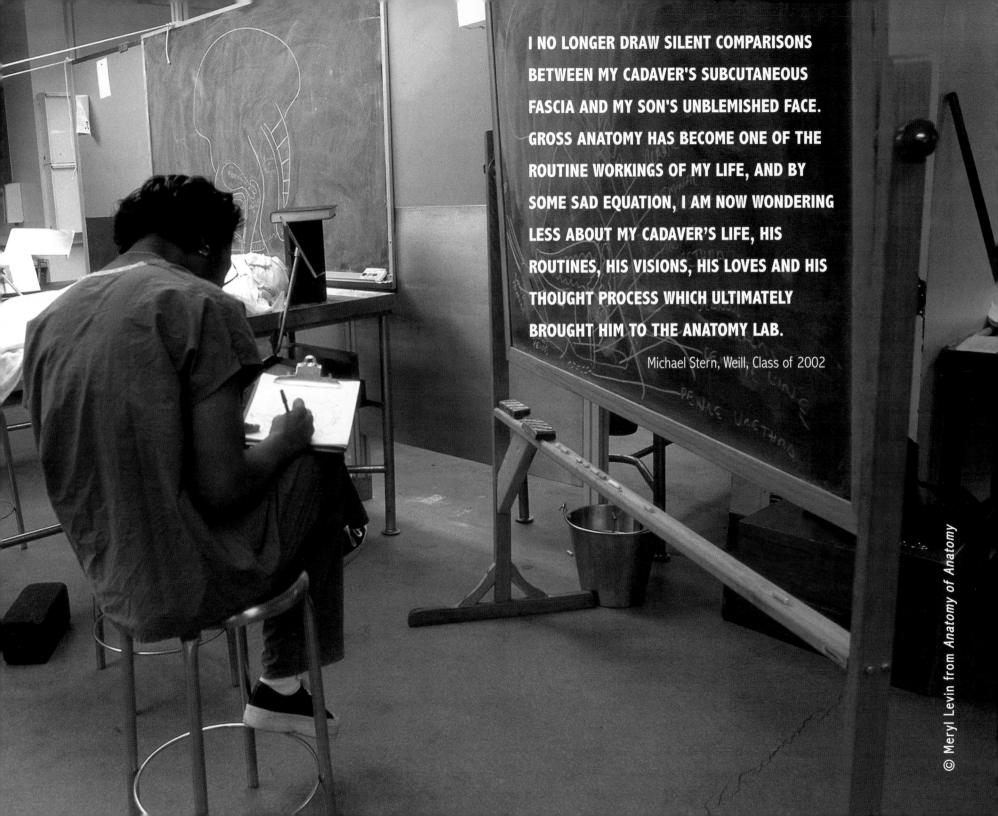

I NO LONGER DRAW SILENT COMPARISONS BETWEEN MY CADAVER'S SUBCUTANEOUS FASCIA AND MY SON'S UNBLEMISHED FACE. GROSS ANATOMY HAS BECOME ONE OF THE ROUTINE WORKINGS OF MY LIFE, AND BY SOME SAD EQUATION, I AM NOW WONDERING LESS ABOUT MY CADAVER'S LIFE, HIS ROUTINES, HIS VISIONS, HIS LOVES AND HIS THOUGHT PROCESS WHICH ULTIMATELY BROUGHT HIM TO THE ANATOMY LAB.

Michael Stern, Weill, Class of 2002

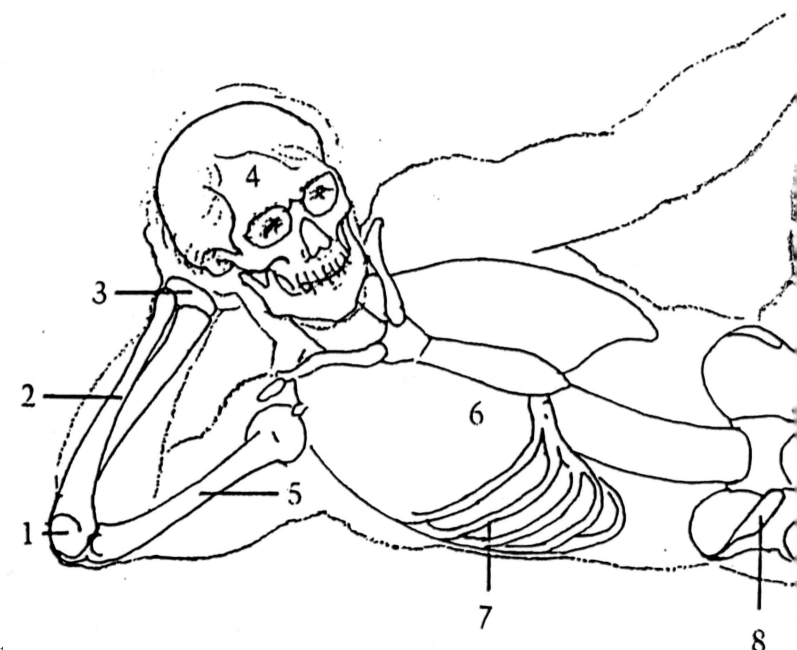

3

2

1

4

5

6

7

8

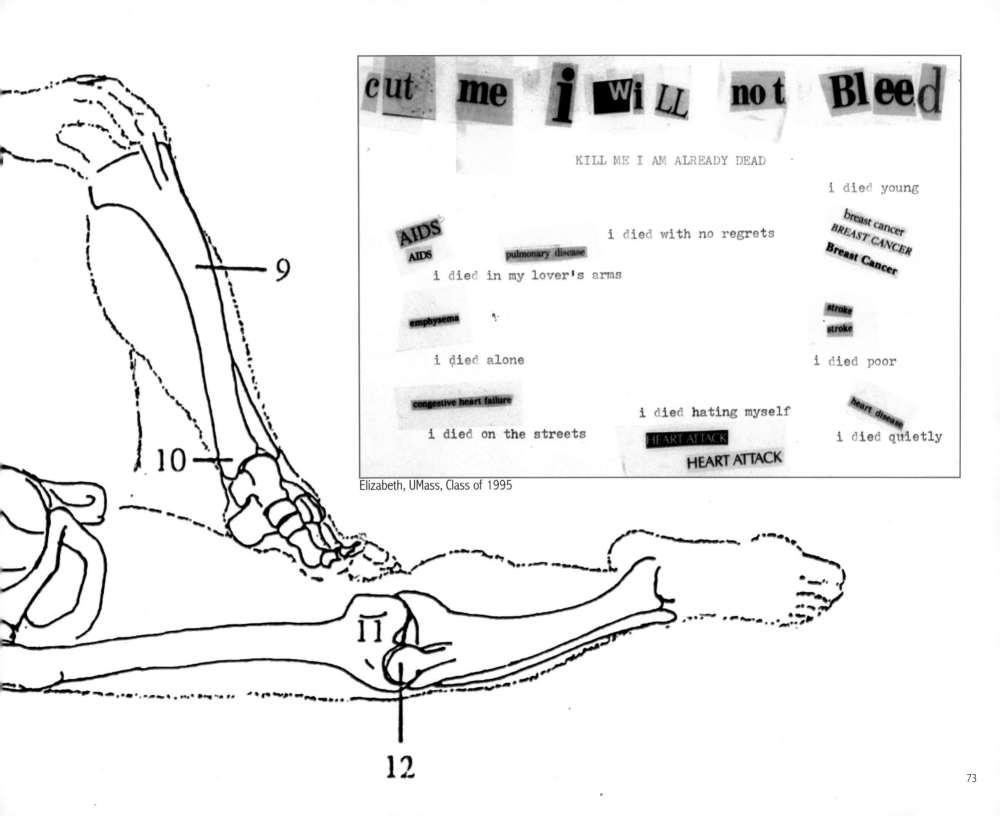

cut me i will not Bleed

KILL ME I AM ALREADY DEAD

i died young

i died with no regrets

AIDS

AIDS   pulmonary disease

breast cancer
BREAST CANCER
Breast Cancer

i died in my lover's arms

emphysema

stroke
stroke

i died alone

i died poor

congestive heart failure

i died hating myself

heart disease

i died on the streets   HEART ATTACK

i died quietly

HEART ATTACK

Elizabeth, UMass, Class of 1995

9

10

11

12

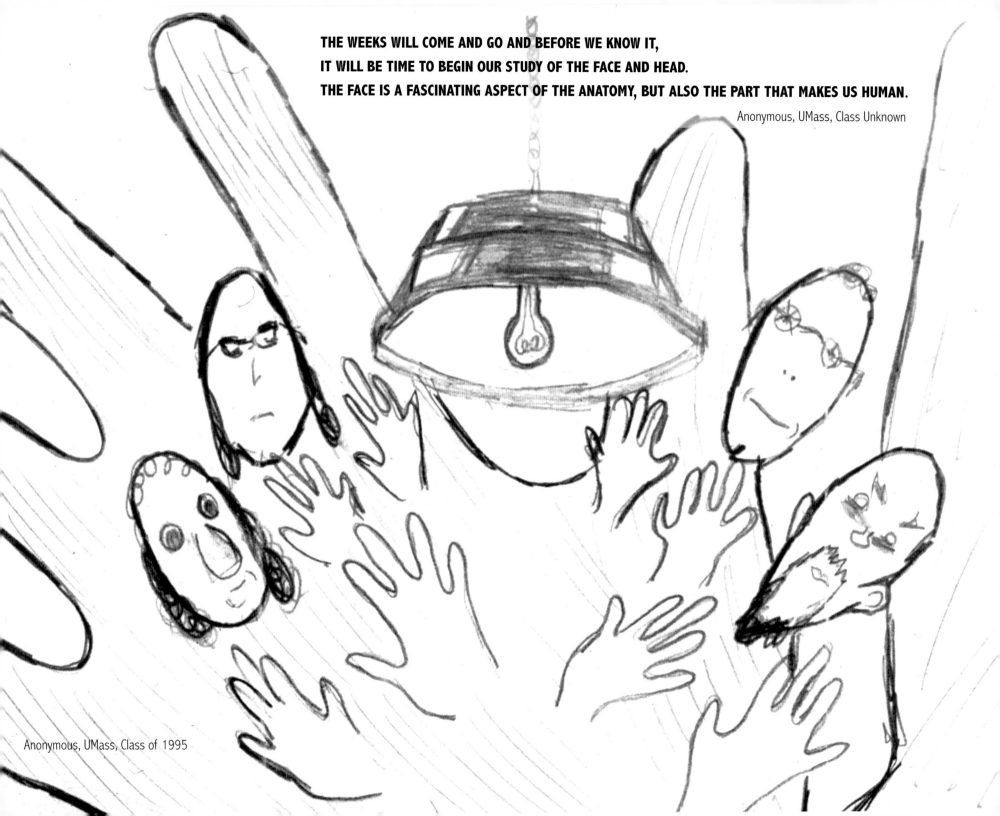

THE WEEKS WILL COME AND GO AND BEFORE WE KNOW IT,
IT WILL BE TIME TO BEGIN OUR STUDY OF THE FACE AND HEAD.
THE FACE IS A FASCINATING ASPECT OF THE ANATOMY, BUT ALSO THE PART THAT MAKES US HUMAN.

Anonymous, UMass, Class Unknown

Anonymous, UMass, Class of 1995

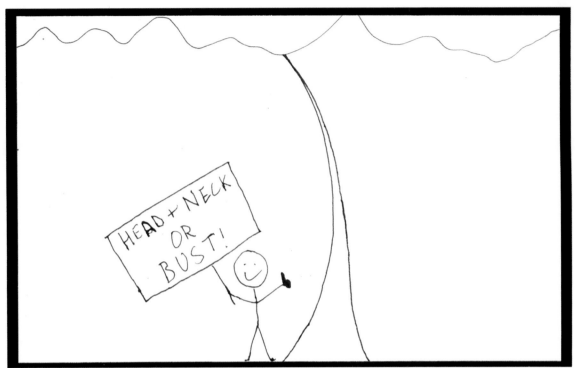

Matt Logalbo, UMass, Class of 2005

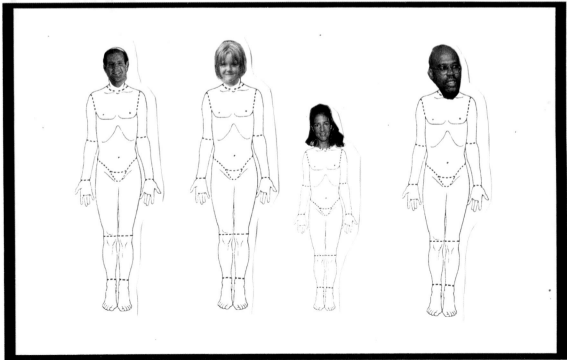

Anonymous, UMass, Class of 2000

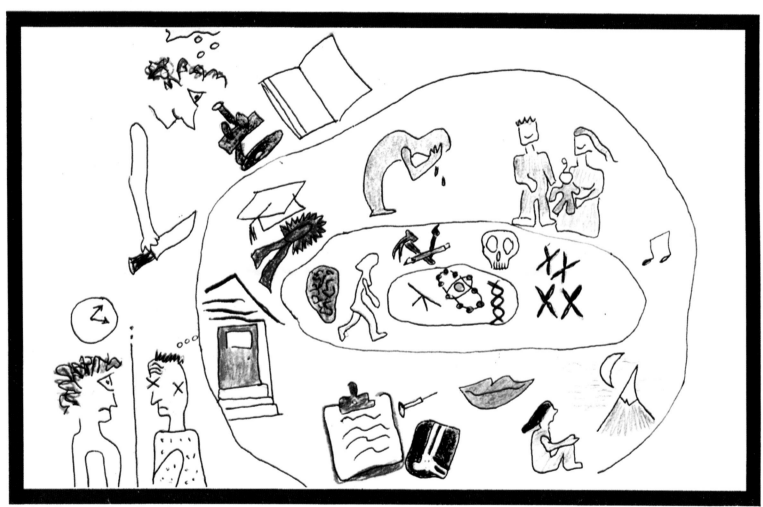

Elizabeth Frutiger, UMass, Class of 2002

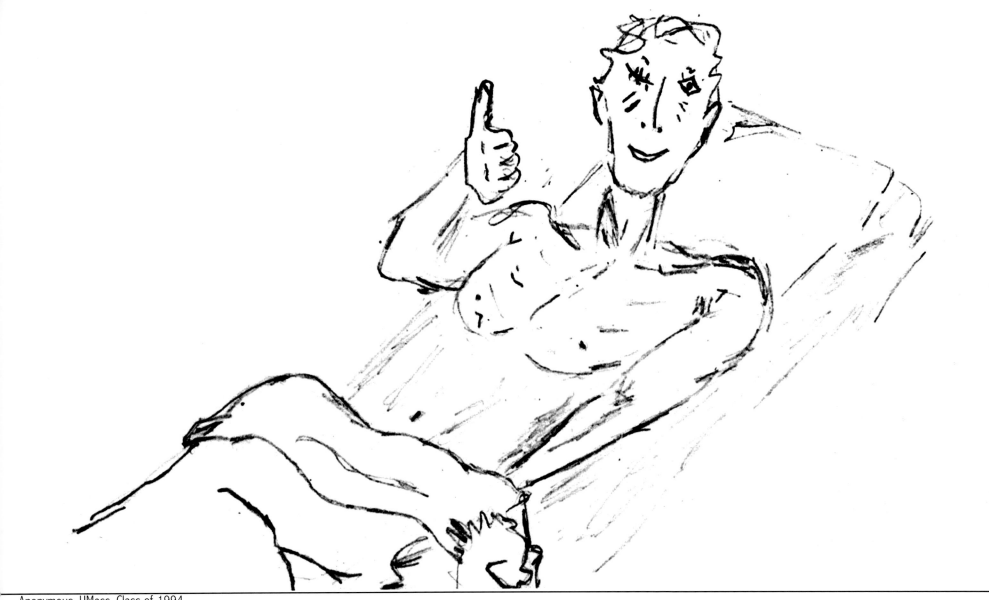

UP UNTIL THIS TIME IT WAS EASY TO IGNORE THE REALITY THAT THIS PERSON USED TO BE ALIVE. . . .

IT MAY SEEM ODD, BUT I FINALLY HAD THE OPPORTUNITY TO MEET MY FRIEND WHO I HAD BONDED WITH OVER THE LAST TWO

MONTHS. IT WAS LIKE MEETING A PEN PAL IN PERSON. I'LL NEVER FORGET DOC, AS WE CALLED HIM.

Anonymous, UMass, Class of 2006

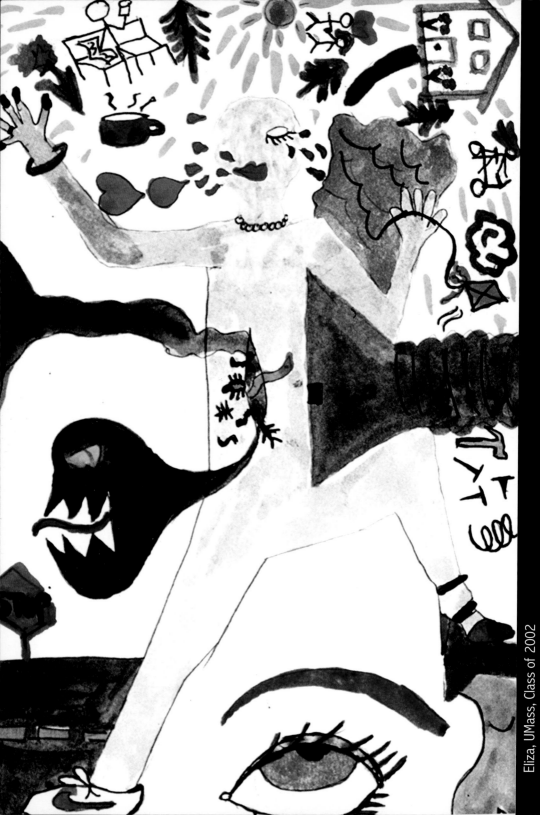

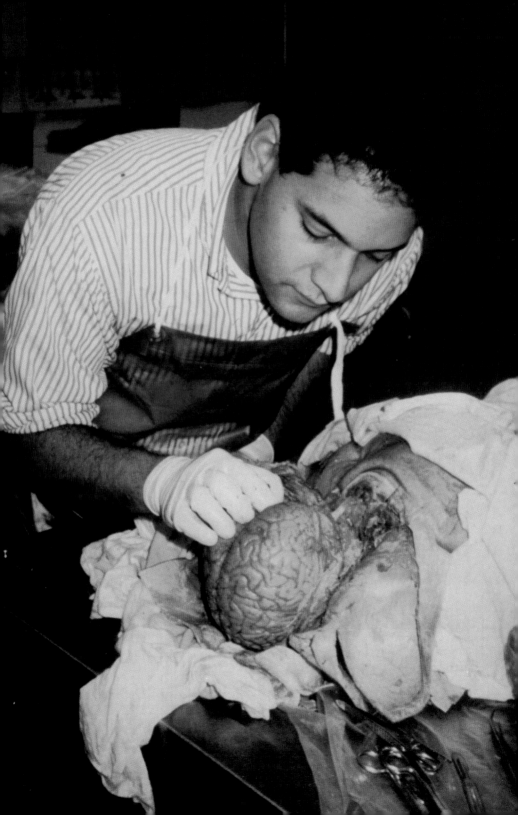

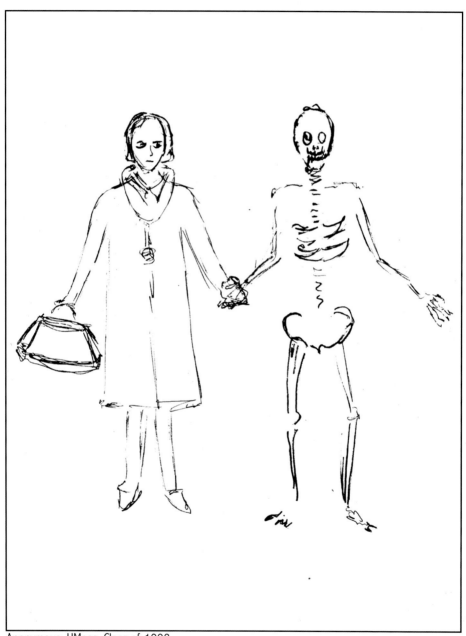

Anonymous, UMass, Class of 1998

WE DID NOT KNOW THEIR NAMES
SO WE NAMED THEM

WE DID NOT KNOW THEIR STORIES
SO WE INFERRED THEM

WE DID NOT KNOW WHAT THEY HAD TO OFFER

(CONTINUED)

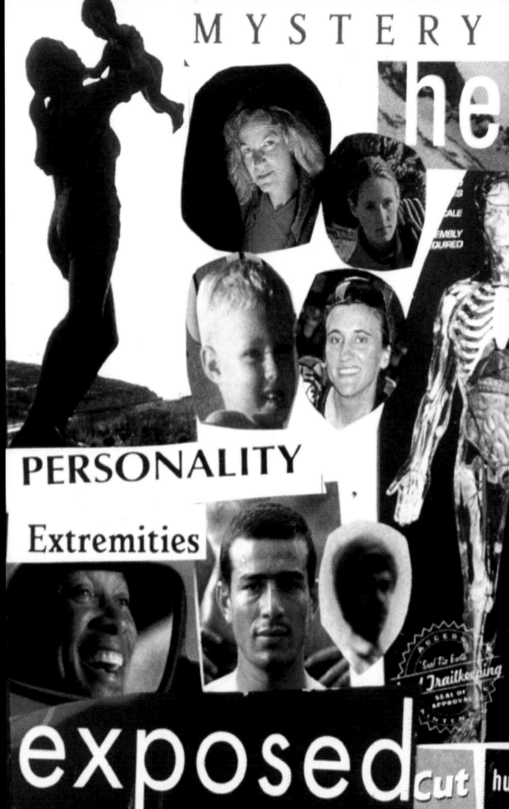

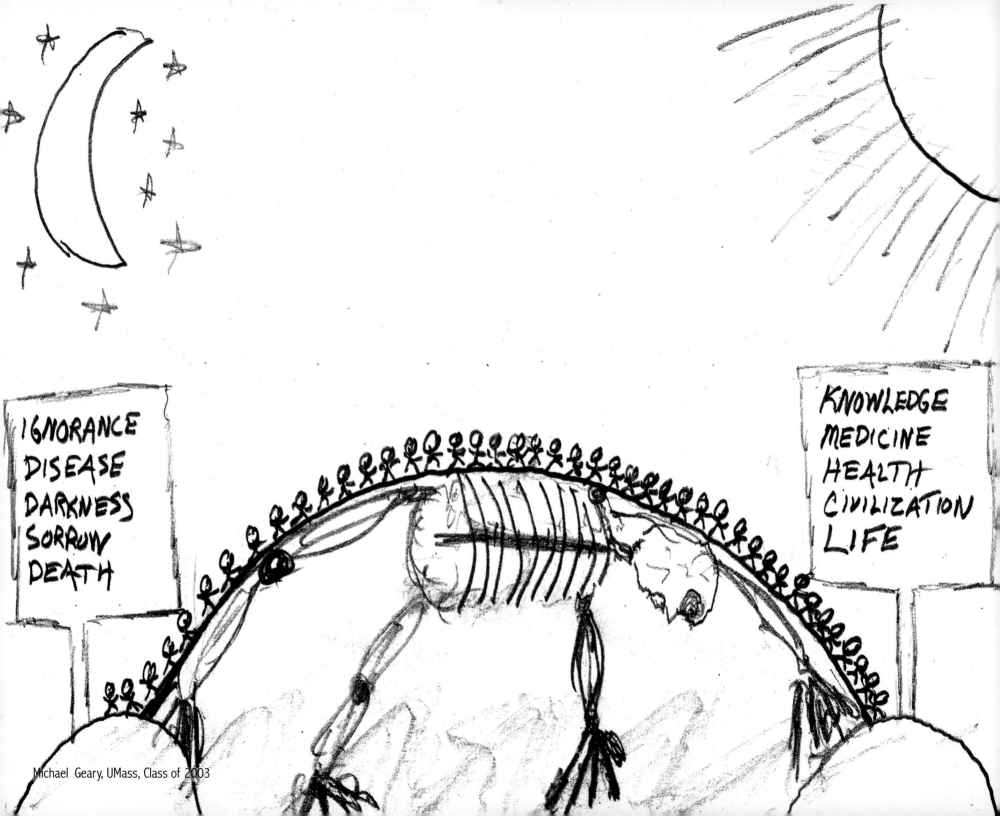

SO WE LEARNED FROM THEM

AND WE WILL REMEMBER THEM.

<small>ALLISON HARGRAVES, UMASS, CLASS OF 2006</small>

In Memoriam...

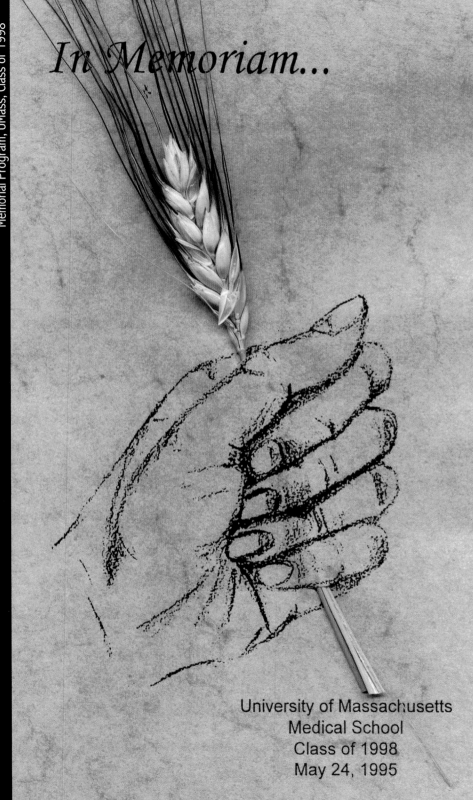

University of Massachusetts
Medical School
Class of 1998
May 24, 1995

SHOW ME THE MANNER IN WHICH A NATION OR A COMMUNITY CARES FOR ITS DEAD AND I WILL MEASURE EXACTLY THE SYMPATHIES OF ITS PEOPLE, THEIR RESPECT FOR THE LAWS OF THE LAND, AND THEIR LOYALTY TO HIGH IDEALS.

BRITISH PRIME MINISTER WILLIAM GLADSTONE

EPILOGUE
REFLECTIONS AND CONNECTIONS

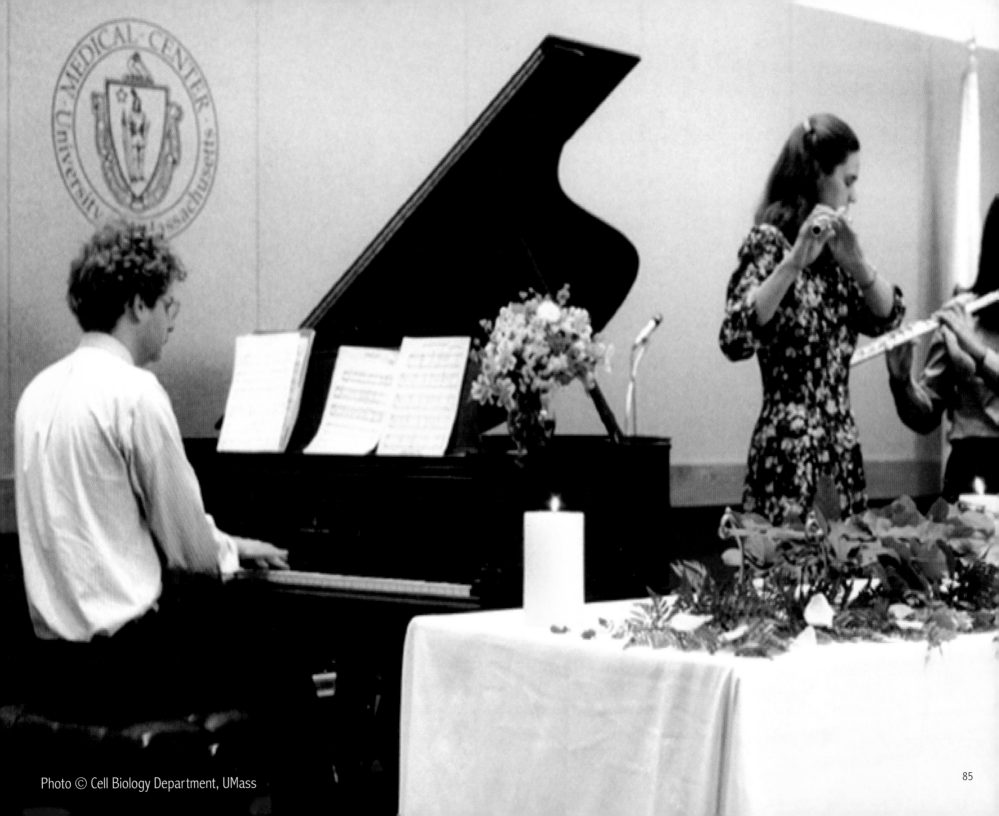

85

The Memorial Services: Student Eulogies for Body Donors and Family Members' Responses

With the completion of the anatomy course, many medical students express the need for additional closure. With painstaking care, students organize and conduct a memorial service in the spring of their first year — an opportunity to publicly acknowledge the gifts they have received from generous and selfless body donors. This gathering serves as a chance for the anatomy students to come together with the families of the body donors, who bid their final farewells to their loved ones.

Traditionally this service is held in May, several months after the anatomy course is completed. It is intentionally timed to coincide with the academic break and also to give the students the needed time and space that allow for a gain in perspective. To their body donors, the students' eulogies express the strong sense of connection and gratitude. You may note that some of the drawings and thoughts in this volume, in response to the anticipating dissection assignment, foreshadow the sense of thanks to the body donor.

Eulogies are a purposeful and consolatory art. In addition to providing comfort for the bereaved families, the medical students express their deep appreciation to the body donors, and in so doing find release for their own emotions. Those assembled learn something about each of the students who compose and deliver these memorable farewells. By conveying their gratitude, the medical students reveal their courage, authenticity and compassion. One can already envision them as future physicians supporting their patients and family members through difficult moments.

This practice affirms that there are creative and spiritual genes in all of us.

Reflections of Medical Students

The following words of a medical student, a personal reflection at one of the memorial services, express with sincerity the confluence of emotions:

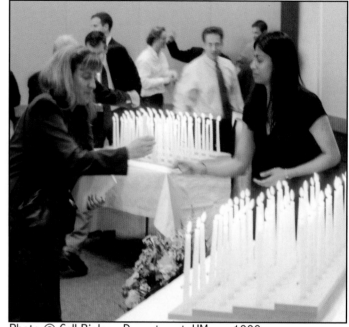

Photo © Cell Biology Department, UMass, 1999

WE REMEMBER SO WELL THAT FIRST DAY: OUR HEARTS POUNDED, OUR MINDS WANDERED, HOW TO DEAL. DAYS PAST, WE FORGOT ABOUT YOU, THOUGHT OF OUR EXAMS, THOUGHT OF ANYTHING, REALLY, BUT YOUR HUMANITY. SO TODAY, FORGIVE US, FORGIVE OUR LAUGHTER, FORGIVE OUR TWISTED FACES, FORGIVE OUR IGNORANCE, FORGIVE OUR DISRESPECT, FORGIVE OUR GROPING HANDS, FORGIVE OUR COLD THOUGHTS, FORGIVE OUR CHILDISH CURIOSITY, AND TOMORROW WE WILL REMEMBER YOU — YOUR PLACID FACE — AND SAY THANK YOU TO ROSE.

Mitch Gitkind, UMass, Class of 1985

The word "cadaver" itself is a distancing, dehumanizing word. For some students, it might be only after the memorial service that they feel "emotionally freed. . . and, more importantly, . . . closure" (Carrie in *Anatomy of Anatomy*, 124). Another student admitted the need to "repress all sentiment" during the course: "The thing in front of you is, indeed, a thing, not a person, not even something that once was a person" (Katie, in *Anatomy of Anatomy*, 126). Only after completing the course is Katie able to attribute personality and kinship to her "first patient." "I think about the cadaver now not as a thing, not as 'my cadaver,' but as 'Alice.'"

So many students eventually personify their cadavers as they express their wonder at the enormity of this very private, intimate, altruistic bequest: >>>

It is never too late to experience the healing power of grief or gratitude, continuing bonds to loved ones, and poignant memories. Many of the students' drawings, shown in this publication, acknowledge that their lives have now intertwined with their cadavers — and that this connection will continue into the future (Figs. 14-17).

WHAT COMPELLED HIM . . . TO SACRIFICE HIS PRIVACY FOR OUR EDUCATION? HE DIDN'T KNOW ME; HE RECEIVED NO PAYMENT FOR HIS WORK. YET HE GAVE ME THE OPPORTUNITY TO EXPLORE EVERY NOOK AND CRANNY OF WHAT HAD ONCE BEEN HIS DOMAIN ALONE. HE GAVE ME THE FREEDOM TO ABANDON MY FEELINGS OF INVASION, AND TO EXPLORE THE SECRETS OF HIS BODY. . . . ERNIE WAS MY TEACHER, AS CLEARLY AS ANY OTHER. HIS TEACHING WAS SILENT, BUT HIS WISDOM ENDLESS. STUDYING HIS BODY PROVIDED AN OPPORTUNITY WHICH ENHANCED MY EDUCATION. BUT IT WAS THE GIVING OF HIS BODY, WHICH HAS REMAINED WITH ME AS A LASTING MEMORY.

Nancy Keene, UMass, Class of 1984

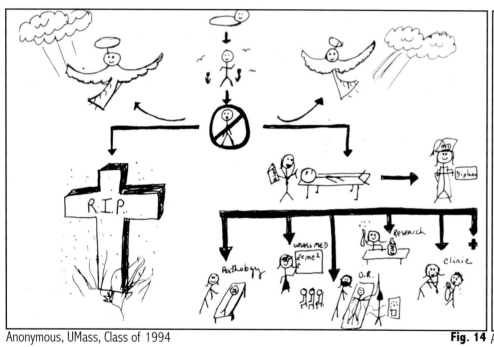

Anonymous, UMass, Class of 1994

Fig. 14

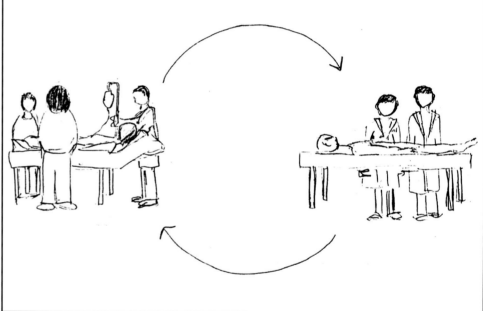

Anonymous, UMass, Class of 2002

Fig. 15

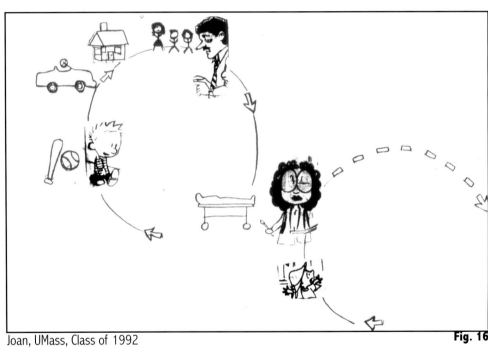

Joan, UMass, Class of 1992

Fig. 16

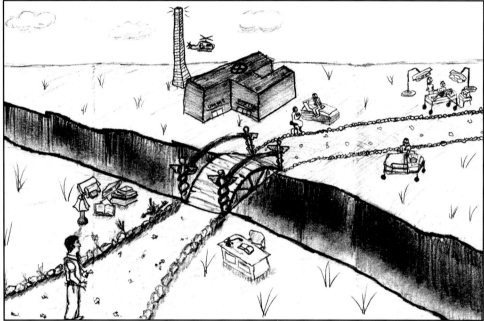

Alex Shushan, UMass, Class of 2003

Fig. 17

FEBRUARY 1999

Established in 1996, the VFW Foundation offers tax and income advantages to those who include the VFW in their Will or Trust. For a free planning kit call 1-816-968-1128.

SUNDAY	MONDAY	TUESDAY	WEDNESDAY	THURSDAY	FRIDAY	SATURDAY
	1 NATIONAL FREEDOM DAY	**2** GROUNDHOG DAY	**3**	**4**	**5**	**6**
7	**8** BOY SCOUTS OF AMERICA FOUNDED (1910) — Last Quarter Moon	**9**	**10**	**11**	**12** LINCOLN'S BIRTHDAY	13
14 VALENTINE'S DAY	15 WASHINGTON'S BIRTHDAY (OBSERVED) / PRESIDENT'S DAY / SINKING OF THE U.S.S. MAINE (1898)	16 NEW MOON	17 ASH WEDNESDAY	18	19	20
21	22 WASHINGTON'S BIRTHDAY	23 FIRST QUARTER MOON	24	25	26	27
28						

Body Donor, Edward Gray

JANUARY 1999
S M T W T F S

MARCH 1999
S M T W T F S

SO . . . YOU THINK YOU'RE HAVING A BAD DAY/WEEK/MONTH/YEAR?

Stephanie (Gray) Siegel, Daughter of Edward Gray

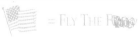 = FLY THE FLAG

Veterans of Foreign Wars

Fig. 18

Family Members' Responses to the Memorial Services

Family members who have attended the memorial services have often written to the students expressing their appreciation for the service.

Dear Class of 2003,

     I have just returned from the Memorial Service held on May 17. Each one of you have given us your first healing. the service was such a balm to our grieving spirits and bodies. Your words, your music, and your present has helped to soothe, and strenghten our lives.

     Thank you.

Some recent classes have asked family members to share photographs, letters, and mementoes about their body donor prior to the memorial service. The daughter of Edward Gray, a talented cartoonist and artist, shared her father's detailed, annotated calendar, which chronicled, alongside his daily cartoons, his daily life and the difficulties presented by his illness — especially the last year of his life (Fig. 18). His daughter appended to the calendar a Post-it: "So . . . you think you're having a bad day/week/month/year?"

In a personal note to the students, she added that she just wished her father had shared with his doctor what he put in his calendar.

Another donor's daughter had trained in anatomy and physiology. In her letter, she acknowledged the joking that went on during her time in the lab as a means of avoiding a focus on the death that surrounded her and her classmates. She recalls two memories that still amuse her:

I LAUGH AT THE CHANEL #5 [PERFUME] THAT WE PUT BEHIND THE EARS OF OUR DEAD CAT [THEY WERE DISSECTING AT THE TIME] IN ORDER TO COVER THE NAUSEATING SMELL OF THE FORMALDEHYDE. AND I REMEMBER THE NAME TAG BEING CHANGED FROM "FRED" TO "FREDERICA" WHEN WE FOUND THE UNBORN FETUS WITHIN HER.

In a serious vein, she, too, needed to share her father's personhood and the details of his death. "He *finally* died the previous May 31, after seven long, tortured years."

As she described many, many personal memories, she realized that, in the process of writing this letter about her father, it became a letter to him:

I fear that we never say 'I love you' to the ones to whom we're closest. I guess all I wanted to say was, 'Daddy, I love you.'

LORI (OSBORNE) ALTOBELLI

Coda: The Web of Life

Finally, in our quest for meaning-making, we marvel at the ability of the human mind to step beyond — to transcend — time and space. Two images, a pencil sketch and a detailed pastel drawing and their accompanying explanations — from two medical students — sum it all up beautifully. In the pencil sketch (Fig. 20), one student examines death and regeneration, and as he expresses it, "the painful truth of our personal demise." He explains the details of his drawing:

An androgynous form is being borne from the ground — the form is a physician that has grown from the knowledge contributed over the generations. Projecting from its face is an eye that emits a ray of light. The ray of light rests on a branch losing a leaf. The light represents a physician's quest for understanding, and the falling leaf represents death. Taken together, I intend a representation of dissection.

Dissection allows physicians to look into the cause of death and to attain a better understanding of medicine. It is a form of regeneration because it perpetuates and builds civilization's base of medical knowledge. The falling leaf decomposes on its descent and begins to merge with other decomposed leaves, eventually creating the collective sustenance from which the physician's form grows. . . .

Thus the cemetery and the physician are both being sustained by the dying leaves. In the upper left hand corner, civilization thrives because of the cycle. The use of natural imagery shows how the human cycle is connected to and must remain in touch with nature. The most sobering of experiences turns into a gracious sacrifice that provides the force behind our perpetuation and progress.

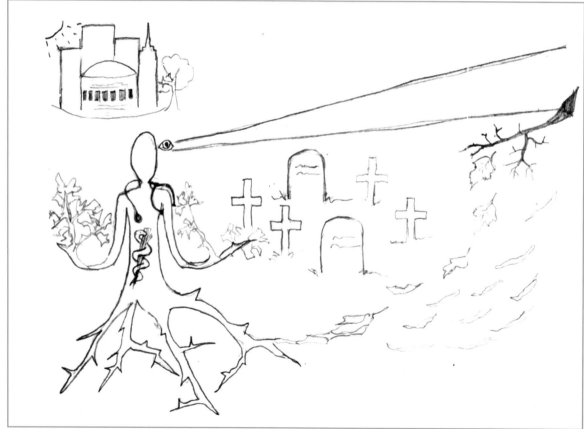

Drawing & Text, Andrew Tzellas, UMass, Class of 2002

Fig. 20

In the pastel image (Fig. 21), another student emphasizes the interconnectedness among peers, faculty, and body donors — past, present, and future.

I depicted the unity and blending of the cadaver and the lab partners, those people who intertwine with him or her and with each other in a quest for understanding. All of the bodies touch and blend and become.

The dissection process is not divorced from nature, for as we undergo this process we create a future that will aid, with compassion, the creatures of the earth. In turn, we help to inspire an ethic of benevolence that will extend through time, and through each other, and across the entire planet.

Dissection blurs time and thus I depict the moon's phases and both day and night. We dissect a person of dignity whose past has led him or her to this place that informs the future. Both the past and the future are held within the moment of cutting and time circles back upon itself. . . . I know that I will be irrevocably altered.

Medical students struggle with comprehending ambiguity, nuance, metaphor, and the inexpressible. Whatever our ethnic, religious, or existential beliefs, we are creatures capable of self-scrutiny and of entertaining the idea of our mortality. The voices of many medical students speak to you in this compilation. They speak from these pages, much the same way that body donors speak to you through the gifts of their bodies.

We are all kin, they tell us. Death is not merely the backdrop against which we play out our morality, but how we come to grips with it is a measure of our humanity.

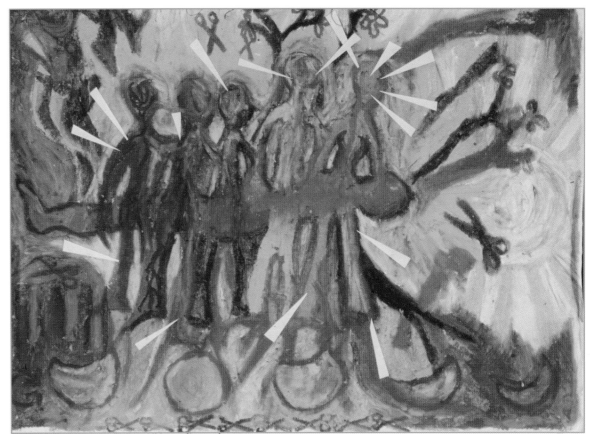

Pastel & Text, Natalie Belkin, UMass, Class of 1997

Fig. 21

REFERENCES

Benjamin, Walter. Aug. 30, 1984. "Healing by the fundamentals." *New England Journal of Medicine* 311:595-597.

Bertman, Sandra. 1997. "From the very first patient to the very last: Soul pain, aesthetic distance and the training of physicians" in Strack S., ed. *Death and the quest for meaning*. Northfield, New Jersey: Jason Aronson.

Bertman, Sandra L. 1991. *Facing death: Images, insights and interventions*. New York: Taylor & Francis.

Gregg, Alan. 1957. *For future doctors*. Chicago: University of Chicago. The epigraph in the Prologue is drawn from this book.

Levin, Meryl. 2000. *Anatomy of anatomy: In images and words*. New York: Third Rail Press.

Marks, SC., Jr, & Bertman, SL.1980. Experiences in learning about death and dying in the undergraduate anatomy curriculum. *Journal of Medical Education* 55:48-52.

Radner, Gilda. 1986. Doctor jokes. http://members.aol.com/parentspage/jokes.html

Chief Seattle's Testimony. 1854. "Humankind has not woven the web of life. We are but one thread within it. Whatever we do to the web we do to ourselves. All things are bound together. All things connect. We are a part of the earth and it is a part of us."

Sharkey, Frances. 1982. *A parting gift*. New York: St. Martin's Press.

Stone, Irving. 1961. *The agony and the ecstasy*. New York: Doubleday.

Zuger, Abigail. July 31, 2007. "A beginning doctor dissects her way toward understanding," *New York Times* review of Christine Montross, *Body of work: Meditations on mortality from the human anatomy lab*. http://www.nytimes.com/2007/07/31/health/31book.html

ACKNOWLEDGMENTS

What started in the mid-seventies as brown-bag lunchtime optional seminars for students, faculty, and staff of the (then) University of Massachusetts Medical Center evolved into a magnificent project. The medical students' courageous willingness to acknowledge their feelings about death and dissection has made this book possible. Many other dedicated people have made valuable contributions: faculty, administrators, staff, body donors, and their family members.

This book is a montage of images and commentaries from different years and presentations. Space does not permit us to include all the student images on dissection that we have been fortunate to receive. Although permission has often been granted to use full names, even then in most cases, only first names and class year have been used to respect the privacy of the contributors. I want to thank all the medical students, whose meaningful, attentive, and provocative responses over the years, catapulted the subjects of death, dying, and bereavement from occasional topics to the mainstream curriculum.

I want particularly to thank the Cell Biology faculty veterans who perspicaciously reviewed many years of material and variations for this module: Sue Gagliardi, Anne Gilroy, Jeanne Keller, Ken Wolffe, Deborah Harmon Hines, Connie Cardasis, and especially John Cooke.

Thank you too to other UMass faculty colleagues, whose feedback as group leaders and many years as facilitators spearheaded the richness and suitability only ongoing revisions could achieve: Bill Damon, Saki Santorelli, Melissa Blacker, Elana Rosenbaum, Betsy Austin, Mel Krant, Peter Viles, Brownie Wheeler, Jay Broadhurst, Mark Quirk, David Hatem, John Zwacki,

and Marjorie Clay. Even the Chancellors and Deans Roger Bulger, Robert Tranquada, John Howe, Jim Dalen, Barry Hanshaw, and Aaron Lazare, often came to the brown-bag lunch sessions, served as group facilitators, and attended the memorial services.

Our Diener, John Santos's steadfast stewardship of the cadavers modeled the dignity that the body donors deserved. He treated the cadavers with such complete respect and reverence. Dianne Person, Administrator of the Anatomical Gift Program, continues to oversee the coordination between body donors, their families, and the medical students with humility and sensitivity in ways that would make Sandy Marks proud.

The computer design skills of Charlene Barron have enriched our presentations over the years, and the vigilance of behind-the-scenes audiovisual competency — beginning with John Ogasion, Barry Davis, Jodi Martineit and most recently, Tom Delaney — were essential to our efforts adding just the needed professional and creative touches.

This project would never have been able to recreate itself so distinctively, year after year, without the tireless labor and attention of administrative staff and assistants: Kathy Olmstead, Rita Wahle, Cary Wyatt McRae, Eileen Siegal Grandstein, Elsie Larson, Betty Flodin, Wendie Allain, Valerie Wedge, Nancy Perkins, and, of course, Hanieh Vahidi and Saeed Sigarodi; or the ongoing encouragement and support of my colleague and friend, Myra Bluebond-Langner.

Many thanks to my current co-collaborator, Meryl Levin, a social documentary photographer whose creativity and talent is matched by her wisdom, humanity, and boundless energy. An anthropologist and a sociologist in examining the dissection course

at Cornell Medical School, she documented a year-long experience in brilliant sensitive photographs and students' journal notations. She generously shared her work, *Anatomy of Anatomy*, with me in both our most recent teaching presentations and in this publication.

Many thanks as well to Digitalclay Interactive, Ltd., and especially to my daughter, Louisa Bertman, for her ability to capture the essence of the amphitheater presentations in the imaginative design of this volume.

To have Jack Coulehan, MD — poet, teacher, clinician, the role model embodiment of the art of medicine and reflective practice — contribute the Foreword is a distinct honor.

Many thanks to Commonwealth Medicine, particularly Tom Manning and Mary Handley, whose ongoing faith in humanities in medicine, resuscitated and supported our program through major curricula and budgetary upheavals, not only at the Medical School but also in our mission of service to hospitals, hospices, and institutions throughout the state and to the public.

Finally, no statement of appreciation can adequately express my indebtedness to Judith Leet, editor par excellence whose skillful and patient insistence on organization and clarity of expression took us to the mat more often than I like to admit.

However impossible our ideas were — or never been done, or outside the box — all the people listed here helped them come to fruition. Thanks also to those unnamed people who simply made our lives easier when the going was hard.

Sandra Bertman is the author of *Facing Death: Images, Insights, and Interventions* (1991), editor of *Grief and the Healing Arts: Creativity as Therapy* (1999), and creator of the DVD and book project *Art, Spirit, and Soul* (forthcoming). At the University of Massachusetts, her teaching career in the departments of psychology (Boston campus) and psychiatry and medicine (Worcester) dates back to 1977. In 1995, for her pioneering work in Humanities and Medicine, and Psychology of Death and Dying, she was one of the recipients of the University of Massachusetts Award commemorating the University's 125 years of service to the Commonwealth for Distinguished Professional Public Service.

Sandra L. Bertman, PhD, FT
Distinguished Professor of Thanatology and Arts
National Center for Death Education Mount Ida College
159 Ward Street Studio Newton, MA 02459
For information, please contact http://www.sandrabertman.com

All proceeds will support the UMass Anatomical Gift Program.